Oil of Life: A Comprehensive Beginner's Guide to Essential Oils

Harnessing the Power of Nature for Everyday Well-Being

Natalie Evans

© Copyright 2024 - All rights reserved.

The content contained within this book may not be reproduced, duplicated or transmitted without direct written permission from the author or the publisher.

Under no circumstances will any blame or legal responsibility be held against the publisher, or author, for any damages, reparation, or monetary loss due to the information contained within this book, either directly or indirectly.

Legal Notice:

This book is copyright protected. It is only for personal use. You cannot amend, distribute, sell, use, quote or paraphrase any part, or the content within this book, without the consent of the author or publisher.

Disclaimer Notice:

Please note the information contained within this document is for educational and entertainment purposes only. All effort has been executed to present accurate, up to date, reliable, complete information. No warranties of any kind are declared or implied. Readers acknowledge that the author is not engaging in the rendering of legal, financial, medical or professional advice. The content within this book has been derived from various sources. Please consult a licensed professional before attempting any techniques outlined in this book.

By reading this document, the reader agrees that under no circumstances is the author responsible for any losses, direct or indirect, that are incurred as a result of the use of information contained within this document, including, but not limited to, errors, omissions, or inaccuracies.

Table of Contents

INTRODUCTION 5

CHAPTER I: The Essence of Essential Oils 7

    Understanding the Extraction Process 7

    Different Types of Essential Oils 11

    Aromatherapy and Its Healing Potential 15

CHAPTER II: Building Your Essential Oils Toolkit 20

    Essential Oils for Beginners 20

    Carrier Oils and Their Role 24

    Tools and Accessories for Safe Usage 28

CHAPTER III: Aromatherapy: Scenting Your Space for Well-Being 33

    Creating a Relaxing Atmosphere 33

    Essential Oil Diffusers and How to Use Them 38

    Blending Oils for Various Moods 41

CHAPTER IV: Topical Applications for Everyday Wellness 47

    Safe Dilution Practices 47

    DIY Essential Oil Blends for Skincare 52

    Massage Oils and Techniques 58

CHAPTER V: Essential Oils for Physical Well-Being 64

    Immune System Support 64

    Managing Aches and Pains 69

    Boosting Energy Naturally 74

CHAPTER VI: Nurturing Mental and Emotional Health 78

Stress Relief and Relaxation 78

Mood Enhancement 83

Sleep Support with Essential Oils 87

CHAPTER VII: Integrating Essential Oils into Daily Routines 92

Creating a Morning Ritual 92

Essential Oils in Self-Care Practices 96

Enhancing Your Evening Routine 99

CHAPTER VIII: Exploring Advanced Blending Techniques 104

Understanding Notes in Essential Oils 104

Crafting Personalized Blends 107

Safety Measures in Blending 111

CHAPTER IX: Essential Oils for Special Occasions 115

Aromatherapy for Celebrations 115

Creating a Relaxing Environment for Guests 118

Using Essential Oils in Meditation and Reflection 121

CHAPTER X: Beyond the Basics: Deepening Your Understanding.. 126

Resources for Further Learning 126

Advanced Applications of Essential Oils 130

Becoming an Informed Consumer 134

CONCLUSION 139

INTRODUCTION

In the embrace of nature's bounty lies the key to holistic well-being, and "Oil of Life" unfolds as a comprehensive beginner's guide to unlocking the therapeutic potential of essential oils. This illuminating book invites readers to embark on a fragrant journey, exploring the ancient wisdom and modern applications of these potent extracts for everyday health and vitality.

The introduction to "Oil of Life" is a fragrant symphony, capturing the essence of essential oils and their profound impact on physical, mental, and emotional well-being. It serves as an aromatic gateway, welcoming both novices and enthusiasts, from curious beginners to seasoned practitioners, into the vibrant world of essential oils, where the natural essence of plants becomes a source of healing and balance.

This book is more than a guide; it is a practical roadmap for harnessing the power of nature to enhance everyday well-being. "Oil of Life" demystifies the world of essential oils, making their benefits accessible to all. From aromatherapy to topical applications, readers are introduced to various uses, empowering them to integrate these natural wonders into their daily routines with easy-to-follow instructions and tips.

The narrative unfolds like a fragrant garden, each chapter a bloom offering insights into essential oils' diverse properties and applications. "Oil of Life" not only delves into the practical aspects of usage but also explores these aromatic treasures' historical and cultural significance, revealing their timeless role in promoting health and vitality.

As the pages turn, readers are guided through the selection, blending, and application of essential oils, creating a personalized journey toward optimal well-being. "Oil of Life" invites exploring the harmony between nature and self-care, where essential oils become potent allies in everyday wellness. Join us on this aromatic odyssey, where the essence of plants becomes the Oil of Life, enriching and elevating the tapestry of your well-being.

CHAPTER I
The Essence of Essential Oils

Understanding the Extraction Process

Essential oils have captivated human senses for centuries, offering a fragrant and therapeutic experience derived from the essence of plants. The extraction of essential oils is a meticulous process that involves harnessing the volatile compounds in various plant parts, such as leaves, flowers, bark, and seeds. This intricate procedure requires a delicate balance of science and artistry, as different plants necessitate distinct methods to yield the purest and most potent essences.

Steam distillation is one of the most common methods employed in essential oil extraction. This ancient technique dates back to the civilizations of Egypt and Mesopotamia, where aromatic plants were distilled for medicinal and cosmetic purposes. Steam distillation involves using steam to rupture the essential oil sacs within plant material, releasing the aromatic molecules. The steam, laden with crucial oil vapor, is then condensed into a liquid, separating the oil from the water. This method is favored for preserving the essential oil's chemical integrity, providing a high-quality product.

Another prevalent extraction method is cold pressing, primarily utilized for citrus fruits. This technique involves mechanically pressing the plant material, usually the rinds of fruits, to release the essential oil. Unlike steam distillation, cold pressing does not apply heat, preserving the oil's delicate aromatic compounds. This method efficiently obtains citrus essential oils known for their bright and refreshing scents, such as Lemon, orange, and grapefruit.

Solvent extraction is employed for plant materials that do not respond well to steam distillation or cold pressing. Commonly used solvents include hexane, ethanol, or supercritical carbon dioxide. The solvent dissolves the essential oil from the plant material, and the resulting solution evaporates, leaving behind the concentrated essential oil. While effective, this method has some drawbacks, as traces of the solvent may remain in the final product, necessitating additional purification steps.

Enfleurage, an ancient method with roots in the perfumery traditions of France, involves placing plant material on a layer of fat or oil to absorb its aromatic compounds. Over time, the essential oil diffuses into the fat, creating a highly fragrant pomade. The process is repeated until the fat is saturated with the essence, and then alcohol is used to extract the essential oil from the fat. Though less common today due to its labor-intensive nature, enfleurage is cherished for its ability to capture the true essence of delicate flowers like jasmine and tuberose.

Supercritical fluid extraction is a more modern method gaining popularity for its efficiency and ability to yield high-quality essential oils. In this process, carbon dioxide is pressurized to a supercritical state, creating a fluid with gas and liquid properties. This fluid is then used to extract essential oils from the plant material. Once the extraction is complete, the carbon dioxide returns to its gaseous state, leaving behind a pure and solvent-free essential oil. Supercritical fluid extraction is particularly advantageous for temperature-sensitive compounds, as it operates at lower temperatures than other extraction methods.

The choice of extraction method depends on various factors, including the plant species, the desired end product, and the aromatic compounds within the plant material. Each technique offers a unique set of advantages and challenges, influencing the quality and characteristics of the resulting essential oil.

Beyond the technical aspects of extraction, understanding the importance of sourcing high-quality raw materials is crucial in producing exceptional essential oils. Factors such as geographic location, climate, and soil conditions significantly impact the chemical composition and aroma of the plants. Ethical and sustainable harvesting practices further contribute to the overall quality of the essential oil, ensuring the preservation of plant ecosystems and biodiversity.

Once the essential oil is extracted, its potential applications are vast. Essential oils are used in aromatherapy, perfumery, skincare, and culinary pursuits. Aromatherapy, the therapeutic use of essential oils, involves inhaling or applying these aromatic compounds to promote physical, emotional, and mental well-being. Essential oils are renowned for alleviating stress, enhancing mood, and even addressing specific health concerns through their antibacterial, antifungal, and anti-inflammatory properties.

In perfumery, essential oils serve as the backbone of countless fragrances. Perfumers artfully blend various essential oils to create intricate scent profiles that evoke emotions, memories, and sensory experiences. Each essential oil contributes its unique aroma, making the perfume a sensory delight and a reflection of the natural world's diversity.

Skincare enthusiasts also benefit from the therapeutic properties of essential oils. These potent extracts often find their way into serums, creams, and cleansers, offering natural solutions for issues ranging from acne to aging. However, it's crucial to exercise caution, as certain essential oils may cause skin irritation or adverse reactions in concentrated forms. Dilution and proper usage guidelines are imperative for safe and effective skincare applications.

In the culinary realm, select essential oils can add depth and complexity to dishes. Whether infusing oils for cooking or enhancing the flavor of beverages and desserts, these concentrated plant essences bring a unique and aromatic dimension to culinary creations. Care must be taken to use food-grade essential oils and to follow recommended dosage guidelines, as the potency of these oils can be overwhelming in large quantities.

In conclusion, the extraction process of essential oils is a fascinating journey that blends ancient wisdom with modern science. Each method contributes to the diverse array of essential oils available today, from the aromatic traditions of steam distillation to the innovative techniques of supercritical fluid extraction. The art of crafting these precious essences extends beyond the laboratory, emphasizing the importance of sustainable sourcing, ethical practices, and a deep respect for the natural world. As we delve into the world of essential oils, we embark on a sensory adventure that enhances our well-being and connects us to the rich tapestry of nature's aromatic treasures.

Different Types of Essential Oils

Essential oils, often called nature's aromatic wonders, represent diverse botanical essences with unique scents and therapeutic properties. These concentrated extracts are derived from various plant parts, such as leaves, flowers, bark, seeds, and roots, through meticulous extraction. Each essential oil type carries its distinctive aroma and therapeutic benefits, making them versatile tools in aromatherapy, skincare, and overall wellness practices.

One of the most popular and versatile essential oils is Lavender (Lavandula angustifolia). Known for its calming and soothing properties, Lavender essential oil is a staple in aromatherapy. Its sweet, floral aroma balances the nervous system, making it an excellent choice for stress relief and promoting relaxation. Lavender oil is also celebrated for its skincare benefits, aiding in healing minor cuts, burns, and skin irritations. Additionally, it is a common ingredient in sleep-inducing blends and natural perfumes.

Peppermint (Mentha × Piperita) essential oil is renowned for its invigorating and refreshing qualities. Peppermint oil's excellent, minty aroma has a stimulating effect on the mind and body. Aromatherapy is often used to combat mental fatigue, enhance focus, and alleviate headaches. When applied topically, Peppermint oil provides a cooling sensation, making it a popular choice for muscle relief and soothing discomfort. Its versatile nature extends to culinary uses, where it can add flavor to beverages, desserts, and savory dishes.

Tea Tree (Melaleuca alternifolia) essential oil is valued for its potent antimicrobial and antiseptic properties. Native to Australia, Tea Tree oil has a medicinal, camphoraceous scent. It is a crucial ingredient in natural skincare products and is known for its ability to combat acne and various skin infections. Tea Tree oil is also used in aromatherapy to promote a sense of cleanliness and freshness. Its antimicrobial properties make it famous for household cleaning solutions and diffuser blends during seasonal illnesses.

The warm and woody aroma of Sandalwood (Santalum album) essential oil has been cherished for centuries. Extracted from the heartwood of sandalwood trees, this oil is known for its grounding and meditative qualities. Sandalwood is frequently used in spiritual and meditation practices to enhance focus and create a serene atmosphere. Sandalwood oil is prized in skincare for its moisturizing and anti-aging properties, making it a luxurious addition to facial care routines.

Eucalyptus (Eucalyptus globulus) essential oil is derived from the leaves of eucalyptus trees and is recognized for its refreshing and invigorating scent. Commonly used in aromatherapy to support respiratory health, Eucalyptus oil helps clear congestion and provides relief during cold and flu seasons. Its antiviral and antibacterial properties make it a popular choice for natural cleaning products, promoting a clean and germ-free environment. Eucalyptus oil is often included in massage blends for its soothing effects on tired muscles.

The floral and citrusy notes of Bergamot (Citrus bergamia) essential oil contribute to its popularity in aromatherapy and perfumery. Extracted from the peel of bergamot oranges, this oil has a bright and uplifting aroma. Bergamot is known for its mood-enhancing properties, helping to alleviate stress and anxiety. In skincare, it is often used to balance oily skin and promote a clear complexion. However, it's essential to note that Bergamot oil is photosensitive, and caution should be exercised when applying it to the skin before exposure to the sun.

With its crisp and citrusy scent, Lemon (Citrus limon) essential oil is a favorite for its refreshing and uplifting qualities. Derived from the peel of lemons, this oil is rich in limonene and is known for its antioxidant properties. Lemon oil is commonly used to boost mood and energy levels in aromatherapy. In skincare, it can help brighten the complexion and address oily skin concerns. Lemon oil is often used in natural cleaning products for its fresh and refreshing aroma.

Chamomile essential oil comes in two main varieties – Roman Chamomile (Chamaemelum nobile) and German Chamomile (Matricaria chamomilla). Both varieties are celebrated for their calming and soothing properties. Roman Chamomile has a sweet and apple-like scent, making it a popular choice for relaxation and sleep-inducing blends. With its deep blue color and warm, herbaceous aroma, German Chamomile is known for its anti-inflammatory and skin-soothing benefits. Chamomile oils are commonly used in skincare and aromatherapy practices to promote a sense of tranquility.

Known for its rich and spicy aroma, Frankincense (Boswellia carterii) essential oil has been revered for centuries in various cultural and religious traditions. Extracted from the resin of the Boswellia tree, Frankincense is often used in meditation and spiritual practices for its grounding and centering effects. In skincare, Frankincense oil is prized for its anti-aging properties, promoting skin elasticity and reducing the appearance of fine lines and wrinkles. Its complex and resinous scent makes it a valuable addition to perfumes and natural incense blends.

Derived from the flowering tops of the Lavandula angustifolia plant, Clary Sage essential oil is recognized for its sweet and herbal aroma. Clary Sage is often used in aromatherapy to alleviate stress, anxiety, and hormonal imbalances. It has a calming effect on the nervous system and is frequently included in blends designed to promote relaxation and emotional well-being. In skincare, Clary Sage oil can be beneficial for balancing oil production and promoting a clear complexion.

Patchouli (Pogostemon cablin) essential oil, with its earthy and musky scent, is derived from the leaves of the patchouli plant. Often associated with the counterculture movements of the 1960s, Patchouli oil has a grounding and balancing effect on the mind and emotions. It is commonly used in perfumery for its long-lasting and distinctive aroma. Patchouli oil is known for its skin-regenerating properties in skincare, making it a valuable addition to products aimed at promoting healthy and radiant skin.

Ylang Ylang (Cananga odorata) essential oil is prized for its sweet, floral, and exotic fragrance. Derived from the flowers of the ylang-ylang tree, this oil is often used in perfumery for its captivating and sensual aroma. Ylang Ylang is also valued in aromatherapy for its mood-enhancing and aphrodisiac properties. In skincare, it can help balance both oily and dry skin types, promoting a harmonious complexion.

Rosemary (Rosmarinus officinalis) essential oil, with its fresh and herbaceous scent, is obtained from the leaves of the rosemary plant. Known for its stimulating and invigorating properties, Rosemary oil is often used in aromatherapy to enhance mental clarity, focus, and memory. It is a popular choice for diffuser blends during study or work sessions. In skincare, Rosemary oil can promote scalp health and encourage hair growth.

These examples only scratch the surface of the vast world of essential oils. The diversity of plants and their aromatic compounds provides an extensive palette for crafting unique blends and addressing various wellness needs. It's important to note that while essential oils offer numerous benefits, they should be used with care. Proper dilution, adherence to recommended usage guidelines, and awareness of individual sensitivities are crucial to ensuring a safe and enjoyable experience with these potent plant extracts.

In conclusion, the different types of essential oils encompass a broad spectrum of aromas and therapeutic properties. From the calming embrace of Lavender to the invigorating freshness of Peppermint, each essential oil holds its unique allure. As individuals explore the world of aromatherapy, skin care, and holistic wellness, these precious plant essences serve as allies on the journey toward balance, relaxation, and vitality. The art of harnessing the essence of plants not only enriches our sensory experiences but also deepens our connection to the natural world and its abundant gifts.

Aromatherapy and Its Healing Potential

Aromatherapy, an ancient practice rooted in aromatic plant extracts, has emerged as a holistic approach to promoting physical, emotional, and mental well-being. The term "aromatherapy" is derived from the fusion of two words: "aroma," referring to the pleasant or distinctive scent of essential oils, and "therapy," signifying a healing treatment. Essential oils, the key components in aromatherapy, are concentrated extracts from various plant parts through meticulous processes like steam distillation, cold pressing, and solvent extraction. The practice of aromatherapy harnesses the therapeutic properties of these essential oils to create a sensory experience beyond mere fragrance.

At the core of aromatherapy lies the belief in the profound connection between scent and emotions. The olfactory system, responsible for our sense of smell, is intricately linked to the limbic system in the brain, which plays a crucial role in emotions, memories, and hormonal balance. When essential oils are inhaled, their aromatic molecules interact with olfactory receptors, sending signals to the limbic system and triggering a cascade of responses. This connection forms the basis for the therapeutic potential of aromatherapy.

One of the primary applications of aromatherapy is in stress management. Essential oils such as Lavender, known for its calming properties, can help reduce stress and anxiety. Inhaling the sweet and floral aroma of Lavender oil induces a sense of tranquility, promoting relaxation and a balanced emotional state. Similarly, with its citrusy and uplifting scent, Bergamot has been shown to alleviate stress and enhance mood. Aromatherapy provides a natural and non-invasive approach to stress relief, allowing individuals to create moments of calm in their daily lives.

Beyond stress reduction, aromatherapy is widely utilized to improve sleep quality. Essential oils like Chamomile, Lavender, and Ylang Ylang possess soothing properties that can help promote relaxation and induce restful sleep. Diffusing these oils in the bedroom or adding drops to a pillow can create a conducive environment for a peaceful night's rest. The calming effects of aromatherapy on the nervous system contribute to improved sleep patterns, making it a valuable tool for those grappling with insomnia or sleep disturbances.

Aromatherapy also plays a significant role in supporting mental well-being. Essential oils such as Peppermint and Rosemary have stimulating properties that can enhance alertness, concentration, and memory. Inhaling these invigorating scents can be particularly beneficial during study sessions or work tasks that require focus. On the other hand, oils like Frankincense and Sandalwood are revered for their grounding and centering effects, making them valuable allies in meditation and mindfulness practices. The ability of aromatherapy to influence cognitive functions highlights its potential as a complementary approach to promoting mental clarity and emotional balance.

The impact of aromatherapy extends beyond emotional and mental realms to encompass physical well-being. Many essential oils possess antimicrobial, anti-inflammatory, and analgesic properties, making them valuable additions to natural healthcare routines. With its potent antimicrobial qualities, tea tree oil is commonly used to address skin infections and support immune function. Eucalyptus oil, known for its respiratory benefits, can be inhaled to ease congestion and promote clear breathing. The versatile nature of essential oils allows for various applications, including massage, topical use, and inhalation, depending on the desired therapeutic outcome.

Skincare is another domain where aromatherapy shines. Essential oils like Rosehip, Carrot Seed, and Geranium are celebrated for rejuvenating and skin-nourishing properties. These oils can be incorporated into facial serums, moisturizers, and cleansers to promote healthy skin and address specific concerns such as aging, dryness, or acne. The sensory experience of applying these aromatic blends contributes to the overall pleasure of skincare routines, creating a holistic approach that addresses both physical and emotional well-being.

Aromatherapy is often integrated into massage therapy to enhance the therapeutic effects of touch. Massage oils infused with essential oils provide lubrication for the massage and deliver the benefits of aromatherapy through skin absorption and inhalation. Lavender, Chamomile, and Clary Sage are popular for relaxation and stress reduction during massages. The combination of tactile and olfactory stimuli creates a synergistic effect, contributing to a more profound sense of relaxation and well-being.

While aromatherapy offers many benefits, it's essential to approach its practice with awareness and consideration. The potency of essential oils requires proper dilution to ensure safe usage, especially when applying them directly to the skin. Some individuals may be sensitive or allergic to certain oils, emphasizing the importance of conducting patch tests and consulting with healthcare professionals, especially those with pre-existing conditions or pregnancy.

Aromatherapy has found its place in various healthcare settings, including hospitals and wellness centers, as a complementary approach to conventional treatments. The soothing scents of essential oils create a more pleasant and calming environment for patients undergoing medical procedures or dealing with chronic conditions. Studies have explored the potential of aromatherapy in reducing pain perception, anxiety levels, and even nausea in medical settings, showcasing its versatility in enhancing overall patient well-being.

As interest in holistic approaches to health and well-being grows, aromatherapy remains a dynamic and evolving field. Ongoing research explores how essential oils exert their therapeutic effects, shedding light on the intricate interplay between scent and the human body. Essential oils, with their diverse aromatic profiles and healing properties, offer a natural and accessible avenue for individuals seeking to enhance their quality of life through sensory experiences and holistic well-being practices.

In conclusion, aromatherapy is a testament to the intricate relationship between scent and healing. From stress reduction to sleep enhancement and mental clarity to skincare, the therapeutic potential of essential oils enriches our sensory experiences and provides a holistic approach to well-being. As we continue to delve into the world of aromatherapy, we embrace the ancient wisdom that connects us to the healing power of nature and the aromatic treasures it offers.

CHAPTER II
Building Your Essential Oils Toolkit

Essential Oils for Beginners

Embarking on the journey into the world of essential oils as a beginner opens the door to a vast and aromatic realm where nature's essences hold the potential to enhance well-being. Essential oils, derived from various plant parts through methods like steam distillation and cold pressing, are concentrated extracts that encapsulate plants' therapeutic and aromatic properties. For those new to essential oils, understanding their basics, selecting appropriate oils, and exploring their diverse applications are pivotal steps in harnessing the benefits of these precious botanical elixirs.

The first step in navigating the world of essential oils is understanding their origins and extraction processes. Essential oils are often extracted from plant leaves, flowers, bark, seeds, and roots, each contributing a unique set of aromatic compounds and therapeutic properties. Steam distillation, a standard extraction method, involves using steam to rupture essential oil sacs within plant material, condensing the resulting vapor into a liquid form. Cold pressing is employed primarily for citrus fruits, mechanically extracting essential oils from the rinds without heat. These methods ensure the preservation of the plants' aromatic and therapeutic integrity, offering users a potent and natural means of holistic well-being.

Choosing suitable essential oils as a beginner involves considering personal preferences, desired effects, and potential applications. With its calming and versatile nature, lavender is an excellent starting point. Its sweet and floral aroma makes it a popular choice for relaxation, stress relief, and promoting restful sleep. Peppermint, known for its refreshing scent, is a go-to for enhancing focus, alleviating headaches, and providing a vital boost. With its potent antimicrobial properties, Tea Tree is valuable for skincare and immune support. As beginners explore the myriad options, they may enjoy experimenting with single oils or blends combining complementary aromas for a more complex sensory experience.

Understanding the various application methods is crucial for beginners seeking to incorporate essential oils into their daily routines. Inhalation is one of the simplest and most immediate ways to experience the benefits of essential oils. Aromatherapy diffusers disperse important oil molecules into the air, providing a gentle and consistent diffusion that can fill a room with the chosen aroma. Direct inhalation, achieved by placing a few drops of essential oil on a tissue or inhaling from the bottle, offers a more concentrated and immediate experience. Adding essential oils to a warm bath or shower can also create a spa-like ambiance and promote relaxation.

Topical application involves diluting essential oils with a carrier oil before applying them to the skin. This method is popular for skincare, massage, and targeted relief. Carrier oils, such as jojoba, almond, or coconut oil, act as a medium to dilute essential oils and ensure safe application. Beginners should be mindful of proper dilution ratios to avoid skin irritation, and a patch test is advisable when trying a new oil. Applying diluted essential oils to pulse points, the soles of the feet, or specific areas of concern allows for absorption into the bloodstream, facilitating their therapeutic effects.

As beginners acquaint themselves with the diverse applications of essential oils, exploring the concept of blending is necessary. Essential oil blends combine two or more oils to create a harmonious and synergistic aroma that can address specific wellness goals. For instance, a Lavender, Chamomile, and Bergamot blend can create a calming and sleep-inducing synergy. Experimenting with different combinations allows beginners to tailor their aromatic experiences to their preferences and needs. The art of blending is both creative and intuitive, offering individuals the opportunity to craft personalized aromas that resonate with them on a deeper level.

Safety considerations are crucial in essential oil exploration, especially for beginners. Essential oils are potent and concentrated, and improper use may lead to adverse reactions. As mentioned earlier, Dilution is a crucial safety practice when applying essential oils topically. Additionally, some oils may be photosensitive and increase the skin's sensitivity to sunlight, requiring caution before sun exposure. Pregnant individuals, nursing mothers, and those with certain medical conditions should consult with healthcare professionals before incorporating essential oils into their routines to ensure safety and appropriateness.

Quality is paramount when selecting essential oils for use. With the growing popularity of aromatherapy, the market is flooded with a myriad of products, ranging from pure and therapeutic-grade oils to diluted or synthetic imitations. Beginners should seek reputable suppliers and brands, prioritizing quality, transparency, and purity. Labels should indicate the botanical name of the oil, its country of origin, and the extraction method used. Essential oils derived from organic and sustainably sourced plants often boast higher quality, as they are free from pesticides and other contaminants.

Education becomes a valuable ally as beginners navigate the world of essential oils. Numerous reputable resources, books, and online platforms provide information on essential oils' properties, uses, and safety considerations. Understanding the chemical composition of essential oils and their interactions with the body fosters a deeper appreciation for their therapeutic potential. Organizations and certification programs dedicated to aromatherapy, such as the National Association for Holistic Aromatherapy (NAHA) or the Alliance of International Aromatherapists (AIA), offer in-depth courses and guidelines for safe and effective use.

The journey into the realm of essential oils for beginners extends beyond individual well-being to encompass the broader concepts of sustainability and ethical practices. Sustainable sourcing ensures the conservation of plant ecosystems and biodiversity, contributing to the long-term availability of essential oils. Ethical considerations involve supporting suppliers who prioritize fair labor practices and community well-being. Conscious consumer choices align with the principles of mindful living and contribute to the planet's overall health.

In conclusion, as a beginner, delving into the world of essential oils is an exploration of nature's aromatic treasures and their potential to enhance well-being. Understanding the basics of extraction, selecting suitable oils, exploring diverse applications, and prioritizing safety are foundational steps in this aromatic journey. Essential oils offer a holistic approach to self-care, allowing individuals to tap into the therapeutic power of plants and create sensory experiences that resonate with their unique preferences and needs. As beginners embrace the art and science of aromatherapy, they open themselves to a world of fragrant possibilities that extend far beyond mere scents, fostering a deeper connection to nature and its innate healing potential.

Carrier Oils and Their Role

In aromatherapy and essential oils, carrier oils are pivotal in crafting a well-rounded and practical toolkit. Essential oils, concentrated extracts from various plant parts, boast potent aromatic and therapeutic properties. However, due to their concentrated nature, essential oils must be diluted before application to ensure safe and optimal use. This is where carrier oils come into play. Carrier oils, also known as base or vegetable oils, serve as a medium to dilute essential oils, facilitating their safe application and providing additional benefits to the skin. Understanding the characteristics, properties, and uses of different carrier oils is vital to building a comprehensive essential oil toolkit that caters to individual preferences and diverse wellness goals.

First and foremost, the choice of carrier oil depends on its intended use and the desired outcome. Popular carrier oils such as jojoba, sweet almond, and coconut oil are often preferred for general dilution and skincare purposes. Jojoba oil, derived from the seeds of the jojoba plant, closely resembles the natural oils produced by the skin, making it an excellent choice for skincare. It is non-greasy, easily absorbed, and provides moisturizing benefits without clogging pores. Sweet almond oil, extracted from almond kernels, is rich in vitamin E and has a light texture, making it suitable for various skin types. Coconut oil, praised for its antimicrobial and nourishing properties, is particularly beneficial for dry or irritated skin.

Argan oil, often called "liquid gold," is another popular carrier oil known for its skin-rejuvenating qualities. Derived from the kernels of the argan tree, argan oil is rich in antioxidants, essential fatty acids, and vitamin E. It is renowned for its ability to moisturize, soften, and improve skin elasticity. The versatility of argan oil extends to hair care, where it can be applied to nourish and tame frizz. Its subtle, nutty aroma adds an appealing dimension to blends and makes it a valuable addition to the essential oil toolkit.

For individuals with sensitive or inflamed skin, the soothing properties of calendula-infused oil make it a gentle and practical choice. Calendula, a vibrant orange flower, is renowned for its anti-inflammatory and skin-calming benefits. Calendula imparts healing properties when infused into a carrier oil, making it suitable for addressing skin irritations, redness, and minor wounds. Calendula-infused oil is often chosen as a base for blends to promote skin recovery and soothe conditions such as eczema or dermatitis.

Grapeseed oil, extracted from the seeds of grapes, is a lightweight and odorless carrier oil known for its astringent properties. Rich in linoleic acid, an omega-6 fatty acid, the skin quickly absorbs grapeseed oil, making it an ideal choice for massage and skincare. Its astringent quality makes it suitable for oily or acne-prone skin, helping to balance oil production. Grapeseed oil is often favored as a base for essential oil blends intended for facial care, contributing to a non-greasy and quick-absorbing texture.

Avocado oil is a rich and nourishing carrier for those seeking an ultra-moisturizing option. Avocado oil, pressed from the pulp of avocados, is abundant in monounsaturated fats, vitamins A, D, and E, and essential fatty acids. Its thick and emollient texture is particularly beneficial for dry or mature skin, providing deep hydration and promoting skin suppleness. Avocado oil is often included in blends designed to address dry skin conditions, support anti-aging efforts, and nourish the hair and scalp.

The unique characteristics of each carrier oil contribute to the overall sensory experience of using essential oils. Fractionated coconut oil, for instance, is a popular choice for its liquid form and long shelf life. It is often used in rollerball blends and massage oils, providing a smooth and non-greasy application. Sweet almond oil, with its mild and slightly sweet aroma, adds a subtle fragrance to blends, enhancing the overall olfactory experience. As individuals explore the world of carrier oils, they may discover personal preferences based on texture, scent, and intended use, allowing them to tailor their essential oil toolkit to their specific needs and preferences.

The role of carrier oils extends beyond dilution and skincare; they also serve as carriers for essential oils in aromatherapy practices. Essential oils are volatile and evaporate quickly when exposed to air. The essential oils are stabilized when blended with carrier oils and have a longer-lasting aromatic presence. This is especially important in applications such as massage or when creating diffuser blends. The carrier oil acts as a vehicle, ensuring that the fragrant molecules of the essential oils are effectively dispersed, allowing individuals to fully enjoy the therapeutic benefits of their chosen basic oil combinations.

In addition to their role as dilution mediums, carrier oils bring their unique benefits to the table. Many carrier oils are rich in fatty acids, vitamins, and antioxidants, offering additional nourishment to the skin. Combining essential and carrier oils in skincare formulations can create synergistic effects, addressing various skin concerns. For example, a blend of lavender essential oil and jojoba oil provides a calming aroma and contributes to skin hydration and balance.

Understanding the individual properties of carrier oils allows for strategic blending to address specific skincare needs. Rosehip seed oil, extracted from the seeds of wild rose bushes, is renowned for its regenerative properties. It is high in vitamins A and C and essential fatty acids, making it a valuable addition to anti-aging blends and formulations promoting skin renewal. Combining rosehip seed oil with essential oils like Frankincense and Geranium can create a potent elixir that supports skin elasticity and reduces the appearance of fine lines and wrinkles.

Carrier oils also play a crucial role in safely applying essential oils to the skin. Undiluted essential oils can be irritating or sensitizing, and proper dilution with carrier oils minimizes the risk of adverse reactions. The recommended dilution ratios vary depending on the individual's age, skin sensitivity, and the essential oil used. Beginners are advised to start with lower dilution ratios and gradually increase as needed, paying attention to how their skin responds.

In aromatherapy, carrier oils contribute to the overall sensory experience. The choice of carrier oil can influence the absorption rate of essential oils into the skin, the aromatic effect's longevity, and the blend's overall feel. Thick and luxurious oils like avocado or coconut may be preferred for a more indulgent and moisturizing experience. In contrast, lighter oils like jojoba or fractionated coconut oil may be chosen for a quick-absorbing and non-greasy application.

As individuals build their essential oil toolkit, it's beneficial to experiment with different carrier oils to find the ones that align with their preferences and desired outcomes. Some carrier oils may be more suitable for specific applications, such as facial serums, body lotions, or hair treatments. By understanding the unique properties of each carrier oil, individuals can tailor their blends to address specific wellness goals and create a personalized aromatic experience that resonates with them on a deeper level.

In conclusion, carrier oils play a multifaceted and integral role in essential oils, serving as dilution mediums and carriers for therapeutic aromatherapy. The diversity of carrier oils allows individuals to customize their essential oil toolkit, catering to individual preferences, skincare needs, and desired aromatic experiences. Whether exploring the soothing properties of jojoba, the regenerative effects of rosehip seed oil, or the lightweight feel of grapeseed oil, the art of blending carrier oils with essential oils enhances the overall journey of well-being. As individuals delve into the aromatic world of essential oils, the careful selection and blending of carrier oils contribute to a holistic and personalized approach to self-care, allowing them to tap into the healing potential of nature and create sensory rituals that uplift the mind, body, and spirit.

Tools and Accessories for Safe Usage

Safe and mindful usage becomes paramount as essential oils gain popularity for their diverse therapeutic and aromatic benefits. Building a comprehensive essential oil toolkit involves selecting a variety of essential oils and carrier oils and acquiring the necessary tools and accessories to ensure safe and practical application. From measuring devices to storage solutions, each accessory plays a crucial role in enhancing the overall experience of using essential oils while prioritizing safety and efficacy.

One fundamental tool for those delving into essential oils is a set of measuring devices. Accurate measurements are crucial when creating blends or diluting critical oils for topical application. Graduated glass droppers and pipettes are commonly used to precisely dispense essential oils, allowing users to control the number of drops added to carrier oils or diffuser blends. Measuring cups or beakers with clear markings facilitate accurate measurements when creating larger quantities of blends. These measuring devices ensure that essential oils are applied in appropriate concentrations, minimizing the risk of skin irritation and optimizing their therapeutic effects.

A dilution chart or guide is another indispensable accessory for safe essential oil usage. These resources provide recommended dilution ratios based on age, skin sensitivity, and the intended use of the essential oil. Dilution charts assist users in determining the appropriate amount of carrier oil to mix with essential oils, promoting safe application on the skin. Beginners, in particular, benefit from referring to dilution guides as they navigate creating personalized blends for massage, skincare, or aromatherapy. Understanding and following these guidelines contribute to a positive and safe essential oil experience.

Regarding topical application, roll-on bottles are practical and convenient tools. These bottles typically feature a rollerball applicator, allowing easy and mess-free application of essential oil blends. Roll-on bottles are trendy for creating personal fragrance blends, applying diluted essential oils to pulse points, or addressing specific skin concerns. The compact size and portability of roll-on bottles make them a versatile accessory for on-the-go aromatherapy and targeted applications, providing users with a convenient way to incorporate essential oils into their daily routines.

A diffuser is a staple tool in the essential oil toolkit, serving as a safe and efficient way to enjoy the aromatic benefits of essential oils. Diffusers disperse important oil molecules into the air, creating a fine mist that can be inhaled for respiratory and emotional well-being. Ultrasonic diffusers use water to disperse essential oils as a cool mist while nebulizing diffusers release undiluted essential oil directly into the air. Diffusers are commonly used in homes, offices, or wellness spaces to create a pleasant and therapeutic atmosphere. They significantly benefit individuals seeking respiratory support, relaxation, or mood enhancement through aromatherapy.

Personal or nasal inhalers provide a discreet and portable option for those who prefer a more direct and localized aromatic experience. These tiny devices typically contain a tube containing a cotton wick soaked in essential oils. Users can inhale through the nasal inhaler, allowing them to enjoy the benefits of essential oils without affecting those around them. Personal inhalers are popular for on-the-spot aromatherapy, offering a quick and convenient way to address specific wellness needs such as stress relief, focus, or respiratory support.

Proper storage is crucial to ensure the longevity and efficacy of essential oils. Dark-colored glass bottles, such as amber or cobalt blue, protect vital oils from exposure to light, which can cause oxidation and degradation of the aromatic compounds. Additionally, airtight seals and dropper caps prevent air from entering the bottle, helping preserve the oils' freshness and potency. Adequately stored essential oils can maintain their therapeutic properties for an extended period, ensuring users benefit from their aromatic experiences.

Labels and labeling tools are essential for maintaining organization and clarity in the crucial oil toolkit. Clearly labeled bottles help users identify and differentiate between different essential oils and blends, preventing confusion and ensuring accurate application. Labeling tools such as waterproof labels, markers, or label makers are valuable for creating professional and durable labels that withstand exposure to oils and moisture. Proper labeling enhances the visual appeal of the essential oil collection and contributes to a safe and organized storage system.

When using essential oils for massage or topical application, choosing the right tools can enhance the overall experience. Massage tools, such as rollerballs or massage wands, facilitate the application of essential oils with a gentle and controlled touch. These tools are handy for self-massage or targeted massage on specific body areas. Incorporating massage tools into the crucial oil toolkit enhances the tactile aspect of aromatherapy, promoting relaxation and providing a sensory-rich experience.

Safety considerations extend beyond applying essential oils to their proper handling and disposal. Essential oils can be potent and may cause skin irritation or sensitization if misused. Gloves of materials resistant to essential oils, such as nitrile or neoprene, protect the skin during blending and dilution. A dedicated set of utensils, such as glass stir rods or stainless-steel spoons, helps prevent cross-contamination when working with multiple essential oils. Adhering to safe handling practices ensures that users can fully enjoy the benefits of essential oils without compromising their well-being.

Educational resources, such as books, reference guides, and online courses, are indispensable tools for individuals looking to deepen their understanding of essential oils. Comprehensive guides provide information on various essential oils' properties, uses, and safety considerations, empowering users to make informed decisions in their aromatherapy practices. Online courses and workshops offer interactive learning experiences, allowing individuals to delve into specific topics, such as blending techniques, aromatherapy for particular health concerns, or advanced essential oil applications. Access to reliable educational resources contributes to developing a well-informed and confident approach to safely and effectively using essential oils.

As individuals build their essential oil toolkit, investing in quality tools and accessories that align with their specific needs and preferences is critical. While a wide range of accessories is available, users can tailor their toolkit to include the tools that enhance their chosen applications and desired experiences. Whether creating custom blends, diffusing aromas, or incorporating essential oils into daily self-care rituals, the right tools contribute to a seamless and enjoyable journey into essential oils.

In conclusion, tools and accessories are indispensable components of a well-rounded essential oil toolkit, enhancing the safety, convenience, and effectiveness of necessary oil usage. Measuring devices, dilution charts, and accurate labeling tools contribute to the precision and organization of blending practices. Diffusers, inhalers, and storage solutions cater to various preferences and applications, allowing individuals to enjoy the aromatic benefits of essential oils in diverse settings. As users explore the multifaceted world of essential oils, carefully selecting and utilizing tools and accessories contribute to a holistic and enriching experience, ensuring that the journey into aromatherapy is enjoyable but also safe and informed.

CHAPTER III
Aromatherapy: Scenting Your Space for Well-Being

Creating a Relaxing Atmosphere

Creating a relaxing atmosphere using aromatherapy is a time-honored practice that harnesses the therapeutic power of essential oils to promote tranquility, reduce stress, and enhance overall well-being. Aromatherapy, derived from the ancient wisdom of plant-based healing, offers a sensory journey that engages the olfactory system and the mind. The deliberate use of essential oils extracted from various plant parts introduces a symphony of scents that can transform any space into a sanctuary of calm and rejuvenation. This essay explores the art and science of utilizing aromatherapy to craft a relaxing atmosphere, delving into the selection of essential oils, application methods, and the impact on the mind and body.

The careful selection of essential oils is central to creating a relaxing atmosphere. Each essential oil has a distinct aroma and unique therapeutic properties that contribute to the overall ambiance. Lavender, with its sweet and floral notes, is renowned for its calming effects, making it a classic choice for relaxation. The scent of Lavender has been shown to reduce anxiety and promote better sleep, making it a versatile and popular option for creating a serene environment. Chamomile, with its gentle and soothing fragrance, is another excellent choice, known for its ability to induce relaxation and ease tension. With its citrusy and uplifting aroma, Bergamot adds a touch of freshness to the mix while promoting a positive mood.

The application of essential oils is equally crucial in creating a relaxing atmosphere. Diffusers are one of the most popular and effective tools for dispersing essential oils into the air. These devices break down essential oils into fine particles, creating a delicate mist that permeates the space. Ultrasonic diffusers, in particular, use water to disperse the oils as a cool mist, maintaining the integrity of the oils' therapeutic properties. Diffusers disperse the aroma and humidify the air, contributing to a comfortable and inviting atmosphere. The gentle hum of the diffuser and the gradual diffusion of aromatic molecules work synergistically to establish a continuous and immersive aromatic experience.

Another effective aromatherapy method is using candles infused with essential oils. Aromatherapy candles, crafted with natural waxes and essential oils, provide a warm and ambient glow while releasing subtle fragrances into the air as they burn. The combination of flickering candlelight and the therapeutic aroma creates a cozy and inviting space, perfect for unwinding after a long day. Soy candles, in particular, are a popular choice for aromatherapy, as they burn cleanly and allow the full aromatic spectrum of essential oils to be released gradually.

Personal inhalers or diffuser jewelry can be employed for a more direct and immediate aromatic experience. Personal inhalers, small tubes containing a cotton wick soaked in essential oils, allow individuals to inhale the aroma directly. This discreet and portable method makes it suitable for creating a relaxing atmosphere. Diffuser jewelry, such as necklaces or bracelets with absorbent pads, provides a stylish way to carry soothing scents throughout the day, allowing individuals to enjoy the calming effects of essential oils wherever they are.

In addition to inhalation methods, topical application can create a relaxing atmosphere. Aromatherapy massage, using diluted essential oils on the skin, combines the benefits of touch with the therapeutic effects of aroma. Essential oils like jojoba or sweet almond oil can be added to carrier oils for a soothing and moisturizing massage experience. This application method contributes to the body's overall relaxation and allows the skin to absorb the beneficial properties of the essential oils, enhancing the holistic well-being experience.

Aromatherapy baths provide yet another avenue for creating a tranquil atmosphere. Adding a few drops of essential oils to a warm bath creates a sensory haven that promotes relaxation and stress relief. The steam from the tub carries the aromatic molecules, allowing individuals to inhale the calming scents while the skin absorbs the oils. Popular choices for bath aromatherapy include Lavender for its calming effects, Eucalyptus for respiratory support, and Ylang Ylang for its floral and exotic notes. The ritual of an aromatherapy bath becomes a therapeutic self-care practice, inviting individuals to immerse themselves in a moment of serenity.

Beyond the immediate sensory experience, the impact of aromatherapy on the mind and body contributes significantly to creating a relaxing atmosphere. The olfactory system, responsible for the sense of smell, is intricately linked to the limbic system in the brain, which regulates emotions, memories, and stress responses. When essential oils are inhaled, their aromatic molecules stimulate olfactory receptors, sending signals to the limbic system and influencing emotional and physiological responses. This direct connection between scent and the brain forms the foundation for the therapeutic potential of aromatherapy in inducing relaxation.

Studies have shown that specific essential oils have measurable effects on physiological parameters associated with relaxation. Inhalation of Lavender essential oil, for instance, has been found to reduce heart rate, blood pressure, and cortisol levels – all indicators of the body's stress response. The calming and soothing properties of Lavender make it a powerful ally in promoting relaxation and creating a peaceful atmosphere. Similarly, the scent of Chamomile has been linked to reduced anxiety levels and improved mood, making it a practical choice for inducing a sense of tranquility.

The impact of aromatherapy on emotions extends to its role in improving sleep quality. Creating a relaxing atmosphere in the bedroom using calming essential oils can contribute to a restful night's sleep. Essential oils like Lavender, Chamomile, and Bergamot have been studied for their sleep-inducing effects. Diffusing these oils in the bedroom or adding a few drops to a pillow creates a sleep-conducive environment, helping individuals unwind and transition into a more relaxed state before bedtime. The gentle and natural aromatherapy approach aligns with healthy sleep hygiene practices, offering an alternative to pharmaceutical sleep aids.

In addition to its effects on the mind, aromatherapy can have physical benefits that contribute to the overall relaxation of the body. Essential oils with anti-inflammatory, analgesic, and muscle-relaxant properties can be incorporated into massage oils or topical blends to address tension and discomfort. Oils like Peppermint, Eucalyptus, or Frankincense are known for their potential to ease muscle tension and soothe aches. Combining tactile massage and the aromatic release of essential oils creates a holistic and therapeutic experience, promoting physical and mental relaxation.

It's important to note that the efficacy of aromatherapy in creating a relaxing atmosphere is subjective and varies from person to person. Individual preferences, sensitivities, and experiences with specific scents contribute to the overall aroma perception. Therefore, selecting essential oils for relaxation is a personal journey, allowing individuals to explore and discover the scents that resonate with them and contribute to their unique sense of calm.

In conclusion, creating a relaxing atmosphere using aromatherapy is a harmonious blend of art and science, combining the selection of essential oils, thoughtful application methods, and an understanding of the mind-body connection. The therapeutic benefits of aromatherapy extend beyond the immediate sensory experience to influence emotions, stress responses, and even sleep patterns. As individuals explore the world of aromatic wellness, the intentional use of essential oils becomes a powerful tool for enhancing relaxation, fostering a sense of tranquility, and creating moments of rejuvenation amid life's demands. Whether through diffusers, candles, massage oils, or personal inhalers, aromatherapy provides a versatile and accessible means of incorporating the healing essence of plants into daily rituals, inviting individuals to pause, breathe, and immerse themselves in the calming embrace of nature's aromatic treasures.

Essential Oil Diffusers and How to Use Them

Essential oil diffusers are popular and versatile tools that bring the therapeutic benefits of aromatherapy into homes, offices, and wellness spaces. These devices offer a convenient and efficient way to disperse the aromatic molecules of essential oils into the air, creating a fragrant and therapeutic ambiance. Understanding the different types of essential oil diffusers and how to use them optimally enhances the overall aromatherapy experience. Whether through ultrasonic, nebulizing, heat, or evaporative diffusers, each method has unique characteristics, benefits, and considerations that create a captivating and soothing atmosphere.

The ultrasonic diffuser is one of the most prevalent types of essential oil diffusers. This popular choice utilizes ultrasonic vibrations to break down a mixture of water and essential oils into fine particles, releasing a cool mist into the air. Ultrasonic diffusers offer the dual benefits of humidifying the surrounding air while dispersing the aromatic compounds of the essential oils. They are typically equipped with adjustable settings, allowing users to control the intensity and duration of the diffusion. Ultrasonic diffusers are user-friendly, easy to clean, and often feature additional features like LED lights for added ambiance. To use an ultrasonic diffuser, fill the water reservoir, add a few drops of the chosen essential oil or blend, and turn on the device for a gentle and continuous diffusion experience.

Nebulizing diffusers represent a more direct and potent method of essential oil diffusion. These devices do not use water or heat but blow air through a glass chamber, creating a vacuum that draws necessary oil directly from a reservoir. The resulting fine mist of undiluted essential oil is released into the air, providing a concentrated and potent aromatic experience. Nebulizing diffusers are appreciated for maintaining essential oils' purity and therapeutic properties without altering their composition. They are often chosen for therapeutic applications where a more intense and immediate diffusion is desired. Using a nebulizing diffuser involves attaching the essential oil bottle directly to the device, controlling the output with adjustable settings, and enjoying the undiluted and full-bodied aroma that fills the space.

As the name suggests, heat diffusers use heat to evaporate essential oils and disperse their fragrance. These diffusers often come in various forms, such as electric heat, candle-powered, or passive ceramic diffusers. Electric heat diffusers typically have a small compartment where essential oils are placed, and a heating element releases the aroma into the air. Candle-powered diffusers use the heat generated by a candle to evaporate the essential oils. Passive ceramic diffusers are porous and absorbent, allowing essential oils to evaporate slowly into the surrounding air. While heat diffusers are easy to use and affordable, they may alter essential oils' chemical composition due to heat application. Users should monitor the diffusion duration to prevent overexposure and ensure a balanced aromatic experience.

Evaporative diffusers rely on airflow to disperse essential oils into the environment. These diffusers typically consist of a pad or filter that absorbs essential oils and a fan or other air-moving mechanism that releases the aroma into the air. Car diffusers, personal inhalers, and certain types of jewelry fall into the category of evaporative diffusers. A small fan disperses essential oil from a pad in car diffusers, providing a refreshing aroma during travel. Personal inhalers are compact devices with an absorbent wick that users can inhale directly. Diffuser jewelry, such as necklaces or bracelets, often has a porous material that holds essential oils, allowing individuals to enjoy the scents throughout the day. Evaporative diffusers are convenient and portable, making them suitable for various settings and applications.

To optimize the use of essential oil diffusers, several considerations and best practices can enhance the overall experience. First and foremost, choosing the suitable essential oils for the desired effect is paramount. Different essential oils offer varying therapeutic benefits, and selecting oils that align with the intended purpose – whether relaxation, focus, or respiratory support – ensures a more effective aromatherapy experience. Understanding the recommended dilution ratios for specific diffusion methods helps maintain safety and prevent potential sensitivities. Diluting essential oils, especially when using nebulizing or ultrasonic diffusers, ensures a balanced and enjoyable diffusion without overwhelming the senses.

Maintaining cleanliness and proper hygiene of diffusers is crucial for both efficacy and safety. Regular cleaning prevents the buildup of residual oils, preventing cross-contamination and ensuring that the diffuser functions optimally. Depending on the type of diffuser, cleaning methods may include wiping down surfaces, emptying and rinsing water reservoirs, or using specific cleaning solutions recommended by the manufacturer. Diligent maintenance not only prolongs the lifespan of the diffuser but also ensures that the aromatherapy experience remains pure and untainted by accumulated residues.

Understanding the importance of diffuser placement contributes to the effective distribution of aromas throughout a space. Placing the diffuser in a central location allows the mist or vapor to disperse evenly, creating a consistent and enveloping ambiance. Consideration of room size is also essential, as larger spaces may require more than one diffuser to achieve the desired aromatic effect. Experimenting with the duration of diffusion sessions allows users to tailor the experience to their preferences, whether they seek a brief burst of aroma or a more prolonged diffusion for an extended ambiance.

Considering the unique characteristics of each diffuser type informs the choice of device for specific preferences and needs. Nebulizing diffusers are ideal for therapeutic purposes, while ultrasonic diffusers suit everyday relaxation. Heat diffusers may be preferable in colder climates, offering a comforting warmth along with the aroma. Evaporative diffusers provide on-the-go convenience and personalization. The variety of diffuser options empowers users to curate their aromatherapy experience based on personal preferences and the desired impact on mood and well-being.

In conclusion, essential oil diffusers serve as indispensable tools in aromatherapy, offering a range of options to cater to diverse preferences and applications. Whether through the gentle mist of ultrasonic diffusers, the concentrated release of nebulizing diffusers, the comforting warmth of heat diffusers, or the portability of evaporative diffusers, each method provides a unique way to enjoy the therapeutic benefits of essential oils. By understanding the characteristics of different diffusers and adopting best practices, individuals can harness the power of aromatherapy to create inviting and soothing atmospheres, fostering relaxation, mindfulness, and a heightened sense of well-being.

Blending Oils for Various Moods

Blending essential oils for various moods is a captivating aspect of aromatherapy, allowing individuals to craft personalized aromatic experiences that align with their emotions, intentions, and well-being goals. Essential oils, derived from the aromatic compounds of plants, possess unique scents and therapeutic properties that can influence mood and emotions. The process of blending oils involves combining different essential oils to create harmonious aromatic compositions that evoke specific feelings or address particular states of mind. Whether seeking relaxation, invigoration, or emotional balance, the thoughtful combination of essential oils opens a sensory gateway to enhance one's dynamic landscape and promote holistic wellness.

Creating a blend that induces relaxation is a popular and cherished aromatherapy aspect. The calming properties of essential oils like Lavender, Chamomile, and Clary Sage make them critical players in relaxation blends. With its sweet and floral aroma, lavender is renowned for its ability to soothe the nervous system and promote a sense of tranquility. With its gentle and herbal scent, chamomile complements Lavender, offering additional calming effects and promoting a restful atmosphere. With its earthy and slightly fruity notes, Clary Sage contributes to relaxation by easing tension and stress. Combining these oils in a balanced blend creates a delightful aroma and provides a powerful tool for winding down, unwinding after a long day, or preparing for restful sleep.

In contrast, blends designed for invigoration and energy often feature citrus and minty essential oils that awaken the senses and uplift the mood. Citrus oils like Grapefruit, Lemon, and Orange are known for their bright and refreshing scents, promoting vitality and optimism. These oils are often included in blends for their ability to uplift the spirits and create a refreshing atmosphere. With its calm and minty aroma, Peppermint adds a stimulating element to the blend, awakening the mind and promoting alertness. With its crisp and energizing scent, Eucalyptus can also be incorporated for its therapeutic properties. Blending these oils in various combinations creates a dynamic and uplifting aroma that can be diffused, applied topically, or inhaled for a quick energy boost.

Emotional balance is a central theme in aromatherapy, and essential oil blends tailored for this purpose often include a diverse range of oils with grounding, harmonizing, and mood-stabilizing properties. Frankincense's rich and resinous scent is revered for its ability to promote emotional balance and a sense of spiritual connection. Lavender, in addition to its relaxing properties, contributes to emotional stability and calm. With its floral and balancing aroma, Geranium is often used to alleviate stress and support emotional well-being. With its citrusy and uplifting notes, Bergamot adds a touch of brightness to the blend, enhancing the overall moving experience. Combining these oils in a well- balanced blend creates a synergistic effect that fosters emotional equilibrium, providing support during stress, uncertainty, or emotional fluctuations.

Blends for focus and concentration are valued in aromatherapy, especially in situations that require mental clarity and cognitive performance. Essential oils for enhancing mental alertness and concentration include Rosemary, Peppermint, and Lemon. With its herbaceous and invigorating aroma, Rosemary has been traditionally associated with memory enhancement and mental clarity. In addition to its energizing properties, Peppermint stimulates mental focus and attentiveness. With its bright and citrusy scent, Lemon is known for its refreshing effect on the mind, promoting mental clarity and concentration. These oils can be blended in various ratios to create a blend that supports cognitive function and aids in maintaining focus during work, study, or any mentally demanding task.

Blending essential oils for stress relief is a common and cherished practice in aromatherapy. Stress-relief blends often feature oils with calming, grounding, and tension-reducing properties. Once again, Lavender takes a prominent role for its versatile calming effects on the mind and body. With its sweet and apple-like scent,

Roman Chamomile is renowned for its ability to alleviate stress and tension. Ylang Ylang, with its exotic and floral aroma, adds a touch of indulgence to the blend while promoting relaxation and emotional balance. With its earthy and grounding notes, Vetiver has a centering effect that helps reduce stress and emotional turmoil. Combining these oils in a stress-relief blend creates a comforting and aromatic oasis, providing individuals with a tool to navigate challenging moments and promote inner peace.

Blending oils for sleep and relaxation is a cherished aspect of aromatherapy, offering individuals a natural and soothing way to unwind and prepare for restful sleep. Lavender, once again, plays a central role in sleep blends for its ability to calm the nervous system and promote relaxation. Roman Chamomile, with its gentle and comforting aroma, enhances the sedative effects of the blend, contributing to a tranquil atmosphere. Sweet Marjoram, known for its warm and herbaceous scent, is often included for its relaxing and comforting properties. With its woody and grounding notes, Cedarwood complements the blend by providing a sense of stability and support for deep relaxation. Blending these oils in a sleep-promoting concoction creates a bedtime ritual that signals the body and mind to unwind, promoting a restful and rejuvenating night's sleep.

Blending essential oils for various moods involves an understanding of each oil's properties and an appreciation for the synergies that can be created through thoughtful combinations. It's critical to consider each oil's top, middle, and base notes to ensure a balanced and harmonious blend. Top notes, such as citrus oils, are light and uplifting, providing an initial burst of aroma. Middle notes, including floral and herbal oils, contribute to the body of the blend, giving complexity and fullness. Like woods and resins, base notes add depth and longevity to the mix, anchoring the overall aroma. Individuals can create blends that unfold over time by combining oils from different categories, providing a dynamic and evolving aromatic experience.

Setting a clear goal or desired mood for the blend is helpful before blending oils. The selection of essential oils for the mix is guided by a specific purpose: anything from stress reduction to sleep promotion, emotional balance, relaxation, invigoration, or focus. Developing a blend that speaks to you personally also requires considering your tastes and unique reactions to other smells. Certain fragrances may have a reassuring or uplifting effect on certain people, while earthy or floral elements appeal to others. People can find their olfactory tastes and make mixes that suit their requirements and preferences by trying and exploring different combinations.

When blending oils, starting with a small batch and experimenting with different ratios is essential to achieve the desired balance. Keeping a record of the ingredients and proportions used in each blend allows individuals to replicate successful combinations and refine their blending skills over time. Additionally, paying attention to the aromatic progression of the blend as it unfolds over time helps in understanding how each oil contributes to the overall experience. This sensory exploration adds an element of creativity and mindfulness to the blending process, allowing individuals to cultivate a deeper connection with the oils and their unique qualities.

Various methods can be employed to blend essential oils, depending on personal preferences and the intended application. A straightforward method is a drop-by-drop approach, where essential oils are added directly to a diffuser or carrier oil, creating a blend in real time. This method allows for immediate adjustments to the blend's composition based on the individual's preferences and sensory experience. Another approach involves pre-blending essential oils in a separate container and allowing the blend to mature over time. This aging process allows the oils' aromatic molecules to meld and harmonize, resulting in a more seamless and integrated blend. Whether blending in small batches for immediate use or preparing larger quantities for future use, the key is approaching the process with intention, creativity, and an openness to the dynamic nature of aromatherapy.

Once a blend is created, various ways exist to incorporate it into daily life. Diffusing the blend using an ultrasonic or nebulizing diffuser allows the aromatic molecules to permeate the air, creating an immersive and therapeutic atmosphere. For a more direct experience, the blend can be applied topically after dilution with a carrier oil, allowing individuals to enjoy the aroma as it interacts with their skin. Massage oils, body lotions, or balms infused with the blend offer a tactile and aromatic experience that enhances relaxation or emotional well-being. A few drops of the blend added to a warm bath create a luxurious and aromatic soak, promoting a holistic sense of tranquility. Personal inhalers or diffuser jewelry provide a portable option for individuals to carry the blend and enjoy its benefits throughout the day.

In conclusion, blending essential oils for various moods is a creative and empowering practice that adds depth and personalization to the world of aromatherapy. The diverse range of essential oils, each with its unique scent and therapeutic properties, provides endless possibilities for creating blends that cater to specific emotions, intentions, and well-being goals. Whether seeking relaxation, invigoration, emotional balance, focus, stress relief, or sleep promotion, individuals can embark on a sensory journey of self-discovery through blending. Selecting, combining, and experiencing different essential oils becomes a dynamic and enjoyable exploration, inviting individuals to tap into the rich tapestry of nature's aromatic treasures to enhance their emotional landscape and create moments of aromatic bliss in their daily lives.

CHAPTER IV
Topical Applications for Everyday Wellness

Safe Dilution Practices

Safe dilution practices in aromatherapy are paramount to ensure that individuals can enjoy the therapeutic benefits of essential oils without compromising their well-being. Essential oils, concentrated extracts from aromatic plants, possess potent properties that can impact the skin, and dilution is crucial in minimizing the risk of adverse reactions. The process involves mixing essential oils with a carrier oil to reduce their concentration before applying them to the skin. Safe dilution practices consider factors such as skin sensitivity, age, and the intended use of the essential oil blend. By adhering to recommended dilution ratios and guidelines, individuals can harness the power of essential oils effectively and responsibly.

One of the fundamental principles in safe dilution practices is recognizing the potency of essential oils. These concentrated extracts contain volatile compounds, contributing to their characteristic scents and therapeutic properties. While this potency is a crucial aspect of their efficacy, it also underscores the need for dilution to prevent skin irritation, sensitization, or adverse reactions. Essential oils are highly concentrated, and their application in undiluted form on the skin can lead to skin reactions ranging from mild irritation to severe sensitization. Dilution provides a controlled and safe way to incorporate essential oils into topical applications, allowing users to experience their benefits without the risk of skin discomfort.

The concept of dilution ratios serves as a guideline for determining the appropriate amount of essential oil to be mixed with carrier oil. Dilution ratios are typically expressed as the number of drops of essential oil per ounce of carrier oil. Common dilution ratios range from 1% to 5%, with 1% being a lower dilution suitable for facial and daily use and 5% for specific applications such as massage or targeted treatments. For instance, a 1% dilution involves adding one drop of essential oil to one teaspoon of carrier oil. In comparison, a 5% dilution entails adding five drops of essential oil to one teaspoon of carrier oil. These ratios can be adjusted based on individual factors, such as skin sensitivity and essential oils.

Understanding skin sensitivity is crucial in determining the appropriate dilution ratio for individuals. Skin types vary; some people may have more sensitive skin than others. Factors such as age, overall health, and pre-existing skin conditions also influence skin sensitivity. Dilution ratios are designed to accommodate these differences and provide a safe and customized approach to using essential oils on the skin. A lower dilution ratio is recommended for individuals with sensitive skin to minimize the risk of irritation. Testing a small amount of the diluted blend on a small skin patch before widespread application helps identify potential adverse reactions and ensures a safe and positive experience.

Age is another significant factor influencing dilution practices, mainly when using essential oils on infants, children, or older people. The delicate nature of a baby's skin requires a higher degree of caution, and essential oils should be used sparingly and at very low dilutions. A 0.1% to 0.25% dilution is generally considered safe for infants, translating to one to two drops of essential oil per ounce of carrier oil. Depending on individual factors, children and older people may tolerate slightly higher dilution ratios, such as 1% to 2%. Adhering to these dilution guidelines ensures that the therapeutic benefits of essential oils can be harnessed safely across different age groups.

The intended use of the essential oil blend also influences the choice of dilution ratio. Different applications, such as massage, skincare, or targeted treatments, may require varying concentrations of essential oils. Massage blends, for instance, often use a higher dilution ratio, typically in the range of 2% to 5%, to accommodate the larger surface area of the body and the prolonged contact with the skin. On the other hand, facial serums or skincare formulations may benefit from a lower dilution ratio, such as 1% or less, to address the sensitivity of facial skin. Understanding the purpose of the essential oil blend allows individuals to tailor the dilution to meet specific needs and optimize the therapeutic effects.

Carrier oils play a crucial role in dilution, serving as a medium to disperse essential oils on the skin. Carrier oils are typically cold-pressed vegetable oils, such as jojoba, sweet almond, coconut, or grapeseed oil, known for their nourishing and emollient properties. When selecting a carrier oil, it's essential to consider factors such as skin type, absorption rate, and potential allergic reactions. The choice of carrier oil can also influence the overall sensory experience of the essential oil blend, as each carrier oil has its unique texture and aroma. Experimenting with different carrier oils allows individuals to find the one that best suits their skin and enhances the application of essential oils.

Common carrier oils used in aromatherapy offer a range of properties to cater to diverse skin types and preferences. Jojoba oil, prized for its similarity to the skin's natural sebum, is suitable for most skin types and absorbs quickly without leaving a greasy residue. Sweet almond oil, with its mild and versatile nature, is well-tolerated by sensitive skin and provides a neutral base for essential oil blends. Coconut oil, known for its moisturizing properties, is solid at room temperature but melts upon contact with the skin. Light and easily absorbed grapeseed oil is suitable for individuals with oily or acne-prone skin. The carrier oil selection can be based on personal preferences, skin needs, and the desired sensory experience.

Once the essential and carrier oils are chosen, the dilution process combines the two components in the appropriate ratio. An amber or dark glass bottle is often recommended for storing the blend, as it protects the oils from exposure to light and helps preserve their potency. To achieve the desired dilution, individuals can use a dropper or a pipette to accurately measure the essential oil drops. Careful mixing or swirling of the blend ensures an even distribution of essential oils within the carrier oil. The resulting diluted blend is ready for use in various applications, such as massage, skincare, or aromatherapy.

In addition to dilution ratios, the frequency of application and duration of use should be considered to maintain safe practices. Essential oils are potent, and continuous or excessive use may increase the risk of sensitization or adverse reactions over time. A cautious approach involves starting with lower dilution ratios, especially for individuals new to aromatherapy, and gradually adjusting based on personal experiences and preferences. Monitoring the skin's response to the diluted blend allows individuals to make informed decisions about the frequency and duration of use, ensuring a positive and safe experience.

Certain essential oils are considered skin irritants or sensitizers; extra care should be taken when diluting and using them. Essential oils such as cinnamon, clove, oregano, and lemongrass are known for their potential to cause skin irritation and should be used in lower dilutions. Phototoxic essential oils, including citrus oils like bergamot, lime, and grapefruit, can cause skin sensitivity when exposed to sunlight. Dilution ratios for these oils should be adjusted accordingly, and individuals should be cautious about applying them before sun exposure. By being aware of the specific properties of each essential oil, individuals can tailor their dilution practices to accommodate potential sensitivities and ensure a safe and enjoyable experience.

Patch testing is a valuable practice in aromatherapy that involves applying a small amount of the diluted blend to a small patch of skin to assess its compatibility. This test helps identify any adverse reactions or sensitivities before widespread application. To conduct a patch test, individuals can apply a small amount of the diluted blend to the inner forearm or a discreet body area. Observing the skin for any redness, itching, or irritation over 24 hours provides valuable information about the individual's tolerance to the blend. The blend can be considered safe for broader use if no adverse reactions occur.

Pregnancy introduces additional considerations in aromatherapy, and safe dilution practices are essential to safeguard both the mother and the developing fetus. While some essential oils are considered safe during pregnancy, others should be used cautiously or avoided altogether. Gentle essential oils such as lavender, chamomile, and mandarin are often recommended for use during pregnancy. In contrast, more stimulating or potentially sensitizing oils like rosemary, clary sage, and basil should be used sparingly and at lower dilutions. Seeking guidance from a qualified healthcare professional or a certified aromatherapist is advisable to ensure that the essential oils chosen and their dilution ratios align with the individual's unique health circumstances during pregnancy.

In conclusion, safe dilution practices in aromatherapy form the foundation for responsible and enjoyable essential oil use. Recognizing the potency of essential oils, understanding individual factors such as skin sensitivity and age, and adhering to recommended dilution ratios are crucial steps in ensuring a positive and safe experience. The choice of carrier oil, the purpose of the blend, and considerations for specific essential oil properties further contribute to the customization of dilution practices. By embracing these principles, individuals can confidently integrate essential oils into their daily routines, harnessing the therapeutic benefits while prioritizing safety and well-being. Safe dilution practices empower individuals to explore the vast and aromatic world of essential oils with mindfulness and intention, fostering a harmonious synergy between nature's botanical treasures and personal wellness.

DIY Essential Oil Blends for Skincare

Incorporating DIY essential oil blends into skincare routines has gained popularity for those seeking natural and holistic approaches to skincare. Essential oils, derived from aromatic plants, possess many therapeutic properties that can benefit the skin. When thoughtfully combined, these oils create personalized blends that cater to individual skin types, concerns, and preferences. DIY essential oil blends for skin care offer a customizable and enjoyable way to enhance the overall health and appearance of the skin, addressing issues such as dryness, acne, aging, and sensitivity. By understanding the unique qualities of various essential oils and their interactions with the skin, individuals can craft effective and nourishing blends that promote a radiant and revitalized complexion.

The first step in creating DIY essential oil blends for skin care is understanding the specific needs and goals of the skin. Different skin types, whether oily, dry, combination, or sensitive, require tailored formulations to address their unique challenges. Additionally, individuals may have specific skincare goals, such as reducing fine lines, promoting an even skin tone, or addressing acne. By identifying these factors, individuals can select essential oils that align with their skincare objectives and work synergistically to promote overall skin health.

Essential oils with moisturizing and nourishing properties are particularly beneficial for those with dry skin. Rosehip oil, extracted from the seeds of the rose plant, is rich in essential fatty acids and vitamins, making it a hydrating and regenerative oil for dry and mature skin. Frankincense essential oil, known for its rejuvenating properties, can help reduce the appearance of fine lines and promote a smoother complexion. With its soothing and balancing effects, lavender oil complements these oils by relieving dry and irritated skin. A simple DIY blend for dry skin could include a carrier oil such as jojoba or sweet almond oil combined with a few drops of rosehip, frankincense, and lavender essential oils.

Conversely, oily or acne-prone skin may benefit from essential oils with antibacterial and astringent properties. Tea tree oil, renowned for its antimicrobial effects, can help combat acne-causing bacteria and reduce inflammation. With its sebum-regulating properties, Clary sage oil helps balance oil production on the skin. Geranium oil, known for its astringent and soothing qualities, adds a floral note while supporting skin health. Crafting a DIY blend for oily or acne-prone skin may involve a lightweight carrier oil like grapeseed or jojoba blended with tea tree, clary sage, and geranium essential oils to create a clarifying and balanced skincare solution.

Combination skin, characterized by oily and dry areas, benefits from a balanced approach that addresses multiple concerns. Essential oils such as chamomile, known for its anti-inflammatory and calming properties, relieve dry and irritated areas. With its balancing effects on sebum production, Patchouli oil helps manage oiliness in specific areas. Lavender oil, versatile in its ability to soothe and nourish the skin, complements the blend by promoting overall skin health. A DIY blend for combination skin could involve a carrier oil like jojoba or almond combined with chamomile, patchouli, and lavender essential oils to create a harmonizing and moisturizing solution.

Aging skin often benefits from essential oils with regenerative and antioxidant properties that support collagen production and protect against free radicals. With its antioxidant-rich composition, Rosemary oil helps combat free radical damage and promotes a more youthful complexion. Carrot seed oil, known for its rejuvenating effects, can enhance skin elasticity and tone. Frankincense oil, prized for its anti-aging properties, complements the blend by promoting cell regeneration and reducing the appearance of wrinkles. A DIY blend for aging skin may include a carrier oil like rosehip or argan combined with rosemary, carrot seed, and frankincense essential oils to create a nourishing and revitalizing skincare solution.

Sensitive skin requires a gentle approach with essential oils with soothing and anti-inflammatory properties. Chamomile oil, mainly Roman chamomile, is renowned for its calming effects on sensitive and reactive skin. With its gentle and balancing properties, lavender oil can relieve skin irritations. Calendula oil, extracted from marigold flowers, adds a soothing and healing element to the blend. Crafting a DIY blend for sensitive skin involves selecting a mild carrier oil such as jojoba or almond, combined with chamomile, lavender, and calendula essential oils to create a calming and nourishing skincare solution.

Once the essential oils are selected based on skin type and skincare goals, the next step is creating a balanced and harmonious blend. Understanding the concept of top, middle, and base notes in aromatherapy is essential for achieving a well-rounded aroma and therapeutic effect. Top notes like citrus oils provide the initial and uplifting scent. Middle notes, including floral and herbal oils, contribute to the body of the blend. Base notes, such as woods and resins, add depth and longevity to the aroma. Combining essential oils from each category allows individuals to create blends that unfold over time, offering a dynamic and enjoyable olfactory experience.

For example, a DIY blend for dry skin could include a top note like bergamot for its uplifting citrus scent, a middle note like rose for its floral and hydrating properties, and a base note like sandalwood for its grounding and moisturizing effects. This combination creates a well-balanced and luxurious blend that addresses the specific needs of dry skin while providing a delightful aromatic experience.

Carrier oils are crucial in diluting essential oils and serving as a medium for their application on the skin. Choosing the right carrier oil depends on individual preferences, skin type, and the desired sensory experience. Lightweight carrier oils, such as jojoba, grape seed, or almond oil, are suitable for facial blends, absorbing quickly without leaving a greasy residue. Decadent oils like coconut, avocado, or shea butter can add moisture and nourish body blends. Experimenting with different carrier oils allows individuals to find the one that best suits their skin and enhances the overall application of the essential oil blend.

Maintaining the proper dilution ratio is crucial to ensure the safety and efficacy of the DIY essential oil blend. Dilution ratios are typically expressed as the number of drops of essential oil per ounce of carrier oil. Common dilution ratios for facial blends range from 0.5% to 2%, while body blends may use ratios between 1% and 5%, depending on the specific application and skin sensitivity. Adhering to recommended dilution guidelines prevents skin irritation and sensitization, allowing individuals to enjoy the benefits of essential oils without compromising their skin health.

Creating a DIY essential oil blend for skincare involves considering the intended application carefully. Facial serums, moisturizers, or facial masks may require different formulations to cater to specific skincare needs. For example, a nourishing facial serum for aging skin could involve a blend of argan oil as the carrier, combined with rosemary, carrot seed, and frankincense essential oils. This concentrated serum can be applied to the face and neck, providing targeted support for mature skin.

Body oils, lotions, or balms offer additional opportunities to incorporate essential oils into skincare routines. Soothing body oil for sensitive skin might include jojoba oil as the carrier, blended with chamomile, lavender, and calendula essential oils. This gentle blend can be applied after bathing to calm and nourish the skin, promoting relaxation and well-being.

Facial steams, a popular skincare ritual, provide an avenue for infusing the skin with the therapeutic benefits of essential oils. Adding a few drops of essential oil to a bowl of hot water creates a fragrant steam that can open pores, promote circulation, and enhance the overall skincare experience. For example, a DIY facial steam for acne-prone skin may involve adding tea tree, clary sage, and geranium essential oils to hot water, purifying and clarifying steam that benefits the skin.

Incorporating essential oils into existing skincare products is another creative way to enhance their efficacy. Adding a few drops of essential oil to a neutral moisturizer, lotion, or unscented base product allows individuals to customize their skincare routine without extensive blending. This approach is convenient for those who prefer simplicity in their skincare regimen while benefiting from the targeted effects of essential oils.

Applying DIY essential oil blends for skin care extends beyond the physical benefits, encompassing a holistic approach that nurtures both the skin and the senses. The aromatic profile of each blend contributes to a sensory experience that can uplift the mood, evoke positive emotions, and create a sense of well-being. Essential oils can engage the olfactory senses, triggering emotional responses and enhancing the skincare ritual. Whether crafting a calming blend for bedtime or a refreshing blend for the morning, the aromatic dimension adds an extra layer of enjoyment to the skincare routine.

In conclusion, DIY essential oil blends for skin care offer a personalized and holistic approach to promoting skin health and well-being. By selecting critical oils based on individual skin type and skincare goals, individuals can create blends that address specific concerns while providing an enjoyable sensory experience.
Understanding the principles of dilution, blending top, middle, and base notes, and choosing suitable carrier oils contribute to the effectiveness and safety of the blends. Whether crafting facial serums and body oils or enhancing existing skincare products, DIY essential oil blends' creative and customizable nature empowers individuals to take an active role in their skincare journey. Through this harmonious fusion of nature's botanical treasures and individual self-care practices, DIY essential oil blends for skin care become a delightful and meaningful expression of holistic well-being.

Massage Oils and Techniques

Massage has been practiced for centuries, serving as a therapeutic and rejuvenating practice that addresses physical and emotional well-being. At the heart of a great massage lies the careful selection of massage oils and the skilled application of various massage techniques. These elements work harmoniously to create a profoundly relaxing and nourishing experience for the recipient, promoting muscle relaxation, stress reduction, and overall balance. Understanding the properties of different massage oils and mastering various massage techniques allows practitioners to tailor their approach to individual needs, creating a personalized and effective massage session.

Massage oils are a crucial component of the massage experience, enhancing the glide of hands over the skin and providing added therapeutic benefits. The selection of the right massage oil depends on the massage's goals, the recipient's preferences, and any specific skin conditions or sensitivities. Sweet almond oil stands out as a popular choice among the widely used massage oils due to its light texture, mild aroma, and nourishing properties. Rich in vitamin E, it moisturizes the skin without leaving a greasy residue. Jojoba oil, known for its similarity to the skin's natural sebum, is another versatile option that absorbs quickly and is suitable for all skin types.

For those seeking a more exotic and indulgent experience, coconut oil offers a tropical touch with its pleasant aroma and moisturizing effects. With its light and non-greasy texture, Grapeseed oil is ideal for massages that focus on relaxation and stress reduction. Additionally, essential oils can be added to carrier oils to create customized blends that cater to specific needs. Lavender essential oil, renowned for its calming properties, can be incorporated for stress relief. In contrast, eucalyptus oil adds a refreshing and invigorating element, making it suitable for massages to ease muscle tension.

Massage techniques play a pivotal role in determining a massage session's effectiveness and overall experience. Various massage modalities cater to different needs, from relaxation and stress reduction to therapeutic and deep tissue work. Swedish massage, one of the most well-known techniques, involves long, flowing strokes, kneading, and circular motions to promote relaxation and improve circulation. It is an excellent choice for those new to massage or seeking a gentle and soothing experience.

Deep tissue massage, on the other hand, targets deeper layers of muscle and connective tissue to address chronic pain and tension. Practitioners use firm pressure, slow strokes, and focused techniques to release tension and promote muscle healing. While deep tissue massage can be intense, it relieves individuals dealing with chronic pain, muscle injuries, or postural imbalances.

Sports massage enhances athletic performance, prevents injuries, and promotes recovery. It incorporates stretching, compression, and specific techniques tailored to the needs of athletes. Sports massage improves flexibility, reduces muscle soreness, and accelerates recovery after intense physical activity.

Shiatsu, a Japanese massage technique, involves applying rhythmic pressure to specific points on the body to balance energy flow or Qi. Shiatsu is deeply rooted in traditional Chinese medicine principles and aims to promote well-being by addressing imbalances in the body's energy pathways.

Thai massage, influenced by traditional Thai medicine and yoga, combines acupressure, stretching, and compression techniques. Practitioners guide recipients through passive yoga-like stretches, promoting flexibility, relaxation, and improved energy flow. Thai massage is often performed on a mat on the floor, and recipients remain entirely clothed.

Hot stone massage incorporates smooth, heated stones placed on specific points of the body and used by the therapist to perform massage strokes. The warmth of the stones enhances relaxation, increases blood flow, and promotes a sense of comfort. Hot stone massage is especially beneficial for individuals seeking deep relaxation and relief from muscle tension.

Aromatherapy massage combines the benefits of massage with the aromatic properties of essential oils. Essential oils are selected based on the individual's preferences and desired therapeutic effects. The massage therapist incorporates the oils into the massage session, enhancing the overall experience with their soothing scents and medicinal properties.

Prenatal massage, tailored for pregnant individuals, addresses the unique discomforts and changes during pregnancy. It utilizes techniques that ensure the safety and comfort of the expectant mother, promoting relaxation and alleviating common pregnancy-related issues such as back pain and swelling.

Reflexology, based on the principle that specific points on the hands and feet correspond to different organs and systems in the body, involves applying pressure to these points to promote balance and overall well-being. Reflexology is a non-invasive and deeply relaxing technique that complements traditional massage approaches.

Effective communication between the practitioner and the recipient is essential regardless of the chosen massage technique. Before the massage session begins, a thorough consultation helps the practitioner understand the recipient's preferences, specific areas of concern, and the desired outcome. This dialogue ensures the massage is tailored to meet the individual's needs and preferences, creating a personalized and satisfying experience.

In addition to the choice of massage oil and technique, the environment in which the massage takes place contributes significantly to the overall experience. Creating a serene and comfortable space involves lighting, temperature, and ambiance. Soft lighting, calming music, and using essential oils for aromatherapy can enhance the relaxation response and contribute to a tranquil atmosphere.

Depending on personal comfort, the actual massage session typically begins with the recipient lying on a massage table, either fully or partially unclothed. A professional massage therapist employs draping techniques to ensure the recipient's privacy and modesty throughout the session. The therapist begins with a warm-up, using gentle strokes and kneading to prepare the muscles for more profound work. As the session progresses, the therapist may adjust the pressure and techniques based on the recipient's feedback and the specific goals of the massage.

During the massage, the therapist focuses on specific muscle groups, addressing areas of tension and promoting relaxation. Effleurage, or gliding strokes, helps spread the oil, warm the muscles, and create a soothing flow. Petrissage involves kneading and compression to release muscle tension and improve blood circulation. Friction techniques, such as cross-fiber friction or circular movements, target more profound layers of muscle and assist in breaking down knots and adhesions. The therapist may also incorporate stretches, joint mobilizations, or passive movements to enhance flexibility and relieve tension.

As the massage session nears its conclusion, the therapist gradually transitions to lighter strokes and effleurage, allowing the recipient to relax. A moment of stillness or gentle rocking may be included to provide a sense of closure to the massage experience. Throughout the session, the therapist remains attuned to the recipient's feedback and adjusts their approach accordingly, ensuring a comfortable and effective massage.

Post-massage care is an integral part of the overall experience. Recipients are encouraged to take their time getting up from the massage table and to drink plenty of water to aid in the elimination of toxins released during the massage. The therapist may offer post-massage recommendations, such as stretches or self-care practices, to prolong the benefits of the massage and support the recipient's well-being between sessions.

Regular massage therapy offers a myriad of physical and mental health benefits. From a physical standpoint, massage helps reduce muscle tension, improve flexibility, and enhance circulation. It can alleviate chronic pain, promote faster injury recovery, and improve musculoskeletal health. Massage also positively impacts the nervous system, promoting relaxation and reducing stress levels.

On a mental and emotional level, massage therapy has been shown to reduce anxiety, improve mood, and enhance overall mental well-being. The release of endorphins, the body's natural feel-good chemicals, contributes to relaxation and contentment. Regular massage can also improve sleep quality, supporting overall health and vitality.

In conclusion, the synergy of massage oils and techniques forms the foundation for a profoundly enriching and therapeutic experience. The careful selection of massage oils based on their properties and the skillful application of various massage techniques allow practitioners to create personalized and practical sessions. Whether seeking relaxation, relief from chronic pain, or targeted therapeutic benefits, the world of massage offers diverse approaches to cater to individual needs. Through the artistry of massage, individuals can embark on a journey of self-care, tapping into the profound healing potential that lies within the hands of skilled practitioners and the transformative power of touch.

CHAPTER V
Essential Oils for Physical Well-Being

Immune System Support

The immune system is the body's intricate defense mechanism, safeguarding against many pathogens and potential threats. Essential oils, derived from aromatic plants, have long been recognized for their therapeutic properties, including their potential to support and enhance the immune system. While not a substitute for proper medical care, essential oils can be valuable additions to holistic wellness practices, offering natural compounds that may contribute to immune system health. Understanding the properties of specific essential oils and their applications provides insight into how these botanical extracts can be incorporated into daily routines to promote overall well-being.

One of the critical aspects of essential oils that makes them supportive of the immune system is their antimicrobial properties. Many essential oils possess natural antimicrobial, antibacterial, and antiviral qualities that can help combat harmful microorganisms. Tea tree oil, derived from the leaves of the Melaleuca alternifolia tree, is renowned for its potent antimicrobial effects. It has demonstrated activity against many bacteria, fungi, and viruses, making it a versatile choice for immune support. Eucalyptus oil, with its distinct aroma, is effective for respiratory issues and exhibits antimicrobial properties, providing a dual benefit for immune health.

Lemon essential oil, extracted from the peels of citrus fruits, is another powerful ally in immune system support. Rich in limonene, a natural compound known for its antimicrobial and antioxidant properties, lemon oil can contribute to a healthy immune response. Its fresh and uplifting scent adds a refreshing element, making it a popular choice for diffusion and aromatherapy practices.

Oregano essential oil, derived from the leaves of the Origanum vulgare plant, is recognized for its potent antibacterial and antiviral properties. The active compound carvacrol, found in oregano oil, has been studied for its ability to inhibit the growth of various pathogens. While oregano oil is highly concentrated and should be used cautiously, its antimicrobial potential underscores its role in immune support.

Clove essential oil, extracted from the buds of the Syzygium aromaticum tree, is rich in eugenol, a compound with antimicrobial and anti-inflammatory properties. Clove oil has demonstrated efficacy against bacteria and fungi, making it a valuable addition to immune-supportive blends. Its warm and spicy aroma adds depth to essential oil combinations for immune system health.

In addition to their antimicrobial properties, certain essential oils exhibit immune-modulating effects, meaning they can influence the activity of the immune system. Frankincense essential oil, derived from the resin of the Boswellia sacra tree, is revered for its immune-supportive properties. Frankincense contains boswellic acids, compounds that have been studied for their anti-inflammatory and immune-modulating effects. The soothing and grounding aroma of frankincense enhances its appeal for both physical and emotional well-being.

Another immune-modulating essential oil is lavender. While commonly associated with relaxation and stress relief, lavender oil also possesses immune-supportive properties. Linalool, a significant component of lavender oil, has been investigated for its anti-inflammatory and immune-modulating effects. The gentle and floral scent of lavender contributes to its versatility in immune-supportive blends, providing a soothing element to the overall aromatic profile.

Echinacea, a well-known herbal remedy for immune support, is also available in essential oil form. Echinacea essential oil is derived from the roots and aerial parts of the Echinacea purpurea plant. It contains compounds such as caryophyllene and germacrene D, contributing to its immune-modulating effects. Echinacea essential oil can be used topically when adequately diluted, offering a convenient and concentrated way to harness the immune-supportive benefits of this traditional herb.

Certain essential oils, such as thyme and cinnamon, are rich in compounds like thymol and cinnamaldehyde, known for their immune-supportive properties. Thyme essential oil has demonstrated antibacterial activity against various pathogens, while cinnamon oil has been studied for its antimicrobial and antioxidant effects. When used judiciously and adequately diluted, these oils can be valuable components of immune-supportive blends.

The application method plays a crucial role in harnessing the immune-supportive benefits of essential oils. Inhalation, either through diffusion or direct inhalation from the bottle, allows the aromatic molecules of essential oils to interact with the respiratory system and the immune cells in the nasal passages. Diffusing a blend of immune-supportive oils in the home or workspace creates an ambient environment that promotes respiratory health and overall well-being. Steam inhalation, where a few drops of essential oil are added to hot water, and the vapors are inhaled, provides a more targeted approach to respiratory support.

Topical application is another standard method for using essential oils to support the immune system. When properly diluted with a carrier oil, essential oils can be applied to specific areas of the body, such as the chest, neck, or soles of the feet. The skin absorbs the beneficial compounds, allowing for systemic and localized effects. This method is particularly effective for essential oils with immune-modulating properties, as they can interact with the immune cells present in the skin.

Massage, incorporating immune-supportive essential oils into carrier oils, offers a dual benefit by combining the therapeutic effects of touch with the aromatic and bioactive properties. A gentle massage using a blend of immune-supportive oils promotes relaxation and contributes to overall immune system health.

Baths infused with essential oils provide a relaxing and immersive way to support the immune system. Adding a few drops of immune-supportive oils to a warm bath allows the aromatic molecules to be inhaled while the skin absorbs the beneficial compounds. This method is especially effective for oils with antimicrobial and respiratory-supportive properties.

Oral ingestion of essential oils is controversial and requires careful consideration and guidance from a qualified aromatherapist or healthcare professional. While some essential oils are considered safe for culinary use and can be added to food or beverages in small quantities, others are highly concentrated and may pose risks if ingested. Caution should be exercised, and thorough research or consultation with a knowledgeable professional is recommended before considering oral ingestion of essential oils for immune support.

When creating blends for immune system support, the synergistic combination of essential oils is often more effective than using a single oil. Blending allows for a broader spectrum of bioactive compounds, enhancing the overall therapeutic potential. A well-crafted immune- supportive blend may include oils with antimicrobial, immune-modulating, and respiratory-supportive properties to provide comprehensive support.

For a diffusion blend that promotes a healthy immune response and freshens the air, consider combining equal parts of tea tree, eucalyptus, and lemon essential oils. This blend offers antimicrobial benefits and contributes to a clean and uplifting atmosphere. Diffuse it regularly, especially during seasons when immune challenges are more prevalent.

For a topical blend to be applied to the chest or soles of the feet, consider combining lavender, frankincense, and eucalyptus essential oils in a carrier oil. Lavender and frankincense contribute immune-modulating effects, while eucalyptus provides respiratory support. This blend can be massaged onto the skin or added to a warm compress for a soothing and immune-supportive experience.

A bath blend for immune system support may include a combination of chamomile, thyme, and tea tree essential oils. Add a few drops of each oil to a carrier oil or an unscented bath gel before incorporating it into the bathwater. This blend supports the immune system and provides a calming and comforting experience.

In conclusion, essential oils offer a natural and aromatic approach to supporting the immune system. Their antimicrobial, immune-modulating, and respiratory-supportive properties make them valuable allies in holistic wellness practices. Whether used through diffusion, topical application, massage, or baths, essential oils provide a versatile and enjoyable means of incorporating immune-supportive benefits into daily routines. As with any wellness practice, it is crucial to prioritize safety, proper dilution, and individual considerations. Integrating immune-supportive essential oils into a holistic approach to well-being can enhance the body's natural defenses and contribute to overall health and vitality.

Managing Aches and Pains

Managing aches and pains is a common challenge many faces, whether due to strenuous physical activity, chronic conditions, or the stresses of daily life. Essential oils derived from aromatic plants have gained recognition for their potential to alleviate discomfort and promote overall well-being. These natural extracts contain bioactive compounds that can offer analgesic, anti-inflammatory, and relaxant effects, making them valuable tools in managing various types of aches and pains. Understanding the properties of specific essential oils and incorporating them into holistic self-care practices provides individuals with a natural and aromatic approach to finding relief.

Lavender essential oil, often celebrated for its calming properties, is renowned for its analgesic and anti-inflammatory effects. The soothing aroma of lavender relaxes the nervous system, helping to ease tension and stress that may contribute to physical discomfort. When diluted and applied topically, lavender oil can relieve sore muscles and joints. Its gentle nature makes it suitable for individuals with sensitive skin, and its versatile application options, such as massage or aromatherapy, make it a popular choice for managing aches and pains.

Peppermint essential oil is another powerful ally in managing discomfort. Rich in menthol, peppermint oil exhibits cooling and analgesic properties that can help alleviate muscle aches and headaches. When applied topically, diluted peppermint oil can create a refreshing and tingling sensation, providing relief. Additionally, inhaling the refreshing scent of peppermint through diffusion or inhalation can contribute to easing tension and promoting a clear and focused mind.

Eucalyptus essential oil, derived from the leaves of the eucalyptus tree, is recognized for its respiratory benefits but also possesses analgesic and anti-inflammatory properties. The active compound, eucalyptol, contributes to its ability to soothe muscle and joint discomfort. Eucalyptus oil can be blended with carrier oil, massaged onto affected areas, or added to a warm bath to create a comforting and therapeutic experience. Its fresh and invigorating aroma enhances the overall sensation of relief.

Chamomile essential oil, mainly German chamomile, is valued for its anti-inflammatory and calming effects. Chamomile contains compounds like chamazulene that contribute to its analgesic properties. Chamomile oil can help ease muscle spasms and joint pain when diluted and applied topically. Additionally, chamomile's gentle and floral aroma has a soothing impact on the nervous system, making it beneficial for managing stress-related aches and discomfort.

Ginger essential oil, extracted from the rhizome of the ginger plant, is recognized for its warming and anti-inflammatory properties. The active compound gingerol gives it the characteristic heat that can help alleviate muscle and joint pain. Diluted ginger oil can be applied topically to areas of discomfort, providing a warming sensation. The refreshing scent of ginger can also be diffused to create a stimulating and uplifting atmosphere.

Frankincense essential oil, derived from the resin of the Boswellia sacra tree, offers a unique blend of anti-inflammatory and analgesic effects. The Boswellia acids found in frankincense contribute to its ability to reduce inflammation and provide relief from discomfort. When diluted and applied to the skin, frankincense oil can offer targeted support for sore muscles and joints. Its resinous and earthy aroma adds a grounding element to the overall experience, making it beneficial for both physical and emotional well-being.

Clove essential oil, extracted from the buds of the Syzygium aromaticum tree, is known for its potent analgesic properties. Rich in eugenol, clove oil exhibits numbing effects that can help alleviate toothaches, muscle pain, and joint discomfort. Due to its intensity, clove oil should be diluted with a carrier oil before topical application. The warm and spicy clove aroma adds a comforting and refreshing aspect to its application.

With its fresh and citrusy scent, Lemongrass essential oil possesses analgesic and anti-inflammatory properties that can contribute to pain relief. Lemongrass oil contains compounds like citronellal and geraniol, exhibiting soothing and refreshing effects. When diluted and applied topically, lemongrass oil can help alleviate muscle aches and joint discomfort. Its uplifting aroma makes it a popular choice for aromatherapy practices that promote relaxation and mental clarity.

Bergamot essential oil, derived from the peel of the bergamot orange, combines analgesic properties with a citrusy and uplifting aroma. Bergamot oil contains compounds like limonene that contribute to its pain-relieving effects. Bergamot oil can relieve muscle tension and discomfort when diluted and applied topically. Its bright and cheerful scent makes it a delightful addition to massage blends or diffuser blends designed for managing aches and promoting a positive mood.

Rosemary essential oil, extracted from the leaves of the Rosmarinus officinalis plant, offers analgesic and anti-inflammatory benefits that can aid in managing various types of discomfort. Rosemary oil contains camphor and rosmarinic acid, which contribute to its ability to soothe sore muscles and joints. When diluted and applied topically, rosemary oil can provide targeted relief. Its herbaceous and invigorating aroma makes it suitable for blending with other essential oils to create synergistic pain relief blends.

Applying essential oils for managing aches and pains involves careful consideration of proper dilution and individual preferences. Topical application, through massage or targeted spot treatments, is a popular and effective method. Essential oils should be diluted with a carrier oil, such as jojoba or sweet almond oil, to ensure safe and comfortable application. The dilution ratio typically ranges from 1% to 5%, depending on the individual's sensitivity and the essential oil used. Applying the diluted blend to areas of discomfort allows the beneficial compounds to be absorbed through the skin, providing localized relief.

Massage is particularly effective for incorporating essential oils into a pain management routine. A soothing massage blend can be created by combining a carrier oil with selected essential oils known for their analgesic and anti-inflammatory properties. The rhythmic application of the blend allows for enhanced absorption and promotes overall relaxation. Whether self-massaging or receiving a massage from a qualified practitioner, the synergy of touch and essential oils contributes to a holistic and therapeutic experience.

Aromatherapy practices, such as diffusion or inhalation, offer an alternative way to enjoy the benefits of essential oils for managing aches and pains. A blend of pain-relief crucial oils in the home or workspace creates an ambient environment that supports relaxation and comfort. Inhalation of the aromatic molecules allows for a direct interaction with the olfactory system, influencing both physical and emotional well-being.

Baths infused with essential oils provide a luxurious and immersive experience for managing aches and pains. Adding a few drops of selected essential oils to a warm bath allows the beneficial compounds to be absorbed through the skin while inhaling the aromatic steam. This method is particularly effective for addressing general muscle tension and promoting overall relaxation. Incorporating Epsom salts into the bath can further enhance the therapeutic effects.

Hot or cold compresses infused with essential oils offer targeted relief for specific areas of discomfort. Adding a few drops of pain-relief crucial oils to a bowl of warm or cold water, soaking a cloth or compress in the mixture, and applying it to the affected area can provide localized comfort. The choice between hot or cold compresses depends on individual preferences and the nature of the pain being addressed.

Creating personalized blends for managing aches and pains allows individuals to tailor their approach to specific needs and preferences. A soothing blend for general muscle discomfort may include lavender, peppermint, and eucalyptus essential oils diluted in a carrier oil for topical application. A blend of peppermint, lavender, and frankincense can be cut and applied to the temples and neck for tension-related headaches. Experimenting with different essential oil combinations allows individuals to discover their preferred blends for various types of discomfort.

In conclusion, essential oils offer a natural and aromatic avenue for managing aches and pains. Their analgesic, anti-inflammatory, and relaxant properties make them valuable allies in holistic self-care practices. Whether applied topically through massage, diffused in the air, added to baths, or incorporated into compresses, essential oils provide versatile and enjoyable options for finding relief. As with any wellness practice, it is crucial to prioritize safety, proper dilution, and individual considerations. Integrating essential oils into a holistic approach to managing aches and pains empowers individuals to tap into nature's botanical extracts' soothing and therapeutic potential.

Boosting Energy Naturally

The quest for sustained energy in our fast-paced world has led many individuals to explore natural alternatives to traditional stimulants. Essential oils, derived from aromatic plants, have emerged as a popular and holistic approach to boosting energy naturally. These concentrated plant extracts contain bioactive compounds that invigorate the senses, enhance mental alertness, and lift natural energy. Understanding the properties of specific essential oils and incorporating them into daily routines allows individuals to harness the revitalizing power of nature without the side effects associated with caffeine or synthetic stimulants.

Peppermint essential oil is a dynamic and energizing oil renowned for promoting mental clarity and alertness. The active compound in peppermint oil, menthol, induces a cooling sensation that can help alleviate fatigue and sharpen focus. Inhalation of peppermint oil vapors through diffusion or direct inhalation from the bottle provides a quick and refreshing pick-me-up. A diluted peppermint oil solution applied topically to the temples, wrists, or back of the neck can contribute to increased energy levels and heightened concentration.

Citrus essential oils, such as lemon, orange, and grapefruit, are celebrated for their uplifting and refreshing qualities. These oils contain compounds like limonene that provide a pleasant and refreshing aroma and stimulate the senses. Diffusing citrus oils in the morning or inhaling their scent during a midday slump can offer a natural energy boost. These oils' bright and citrusy notes create a positive and energizing ambiance, making them popular choices for enhancing mood and motivation.

Eucalyptus essential oil, commonly associated with respiratory benefits, also possesses stimulating properties that can combat fatigue. The refreshing scent of eucalyptus oil clears the mind and promotes alertness. Diffusing eucalyptus oil in workspaces or adding a few drops to a personal inhaler provides a revitalizing experience. Its crisp and camphorous aroma is a natural energizer, making it beneficial for combating mental and physical lethargy.

Rosemary essential oil, derived from the aromatic herb Rosmarinus officinalis, is recognized for enhancing cognitive function and combating mental fatigue. The active compounds in rosemary oil, such as 1,8-cineole, have been studied for their positive effects on memory and mental alertness. Diffusing rosemary oil or inhaling its scent directly can stimulate the mind and promote a sense of wakefulness. This makes rosemary oil a valuable ally for boosting energy during mental exertion or when facing cognitive challenges.

Ginger essential oil, known for its warming and stimulating properties, boosts natural energy by promoting circulation and reducing feelings of sluggishness. The active compound gingerol contributes to its therapeutic effects. Diffusing ginger oil or inhaling its aroma directly from the bottle can help combat fatigue and increase overall vitality. Additionally, a diluted solution of ginger oil applied topically to pulse points or massaged into the skin offers a refreshing and energizing experience.

The uplifting and floral aroma of jasmine essential oil makes it a unique and luxurious option for boosting energy naturally. Jasmine oil is known for its ability to reduce feelings of fatigue and enhance alertness. Inhaling jasmine oil's sweet and intoxicating scent through diffusion or direct inhalation can create a sense of revitalization. The aromatic profile of jasmine oil also carries mood-enhancing properties, making it a delightful choice for infusing a touch of luxury into energy-boosting routines.

With its vibrant and citrusy scent, Lemongrass essential oil is a popular choice for promoting energy and vitality. Lemongrass oil contains compounds like citral that contribute to its stimulating effects. Diffusing lemongrass oil in the morning or adding a few drops to a personal inhaler can provide a natural and uplifting energy lift. The fresh and zesty aroma of lemongrass oil stimulates the senses and adds a touch of brightness to the enviroment.

Essential oils' diverse and energizing effects can be harnessed through various application methods. Diffusion is a popular and convenient way to enjoy the benefits of essential oils throughout the day. An ultrasonic or simple aromatherapy diffuser allows individuals to disperse aromatic molecules into the air, creating an energizing and revitalizing atmosphere in their living or working spaces.

Inhalation directly from the bottle or via a personal inhaler provides a quick and portable method for accessing the energizing properties of essential oils. This approach is beneficial during fatigue or when a natural energy boost is needed. Inhaling the aromatic vapors of selected oils, such as peppermint, citrus, or eucalyptus, can help combat sluggishness and promote a sense of alertness.

When properly diluted with a carrier oil, the topical application of essential oils allows individuals to experience the invigorating effects directly on their skin. Creating a diluted blend and applying it to pulse points, such as the wrists, neck, or temples, enables the absorption of the bioactive compounds. This method effectively sustains a subtle and continuous release of the oils' energizing properties throughout the day.

Creating personalized blends for energy support allows individuals to tailor their approach to specific needs and preferences. A refreshing morning blend may include citrus oils like lemon and orange and a hint of refreshing peppermint. Diffusing this blend in the morning or applying it topically can provide a natural and uplifting start to the day. For sustained energy during work or study sessions, a mix of rosemary and ginger can be diffused or inhaled, offering cognitive support and combating mental fatigue.

In conclusion, essential oils offer a natural and aromatic approach to boosting energy. Their invigorating and stimulating properties provide a refreshing alternative to traditional stimulants. Whether inhaled through diffusion, applied topically, or incorporated into personalized blends, essential oils offer a versatile and enjoyable means of enhancing vitality and alertness. As with any wellness practice, it is crucial to prioritize safety, proper dilution, and individual considerations. Integrating essential oils into daily routines empowers individuals to tap into the energizing potential of nature's botanical extracts, fostering a holistic and sustainable approach to maintaining vitality.

CHAPTER VI
Nurturing Mental and Emotional Health

Stress Relief and Relaxation

Stress has become a prevalent aspect of daily life in our fast-paced and demanding world. Pursuing effective stress relief and relaxation strategies has led many individuals to explore natural alternatives, and essential oils have emerged as powerful allies in this endeavor. Derived from aromatic plants, these concentrated extracts contain bioactive compounds that can positively impact the nervous system, promoting relaxation, reducing stress, and contributing to overall well-being.

Lavender essential oil stands out as a cornerstone in stress relief and relaxation. Renowned for its calming and soothing properties, lavender oil has been used for centuries to alleviate stress and promote relaxation. When inhaled, the active compounds in lavender, such as linalool and linalyl acetate, interact with the olfactory system, signaling the brain to induce a sense of calm. Diffusing lavender oil in the home or adding a few drops to a pillowcase before bedtime creates a serene atmosphere that encourages relaxation and quality sleep. Additionally, diluted lavender oil can be applied topically to pulse points or added to a warm bath for a luxurious, stress-relieving experience.

Chamomile essential oil, particularly the Roman chamomile variety, is another potent oil for stress relief and relaxation. Chamomile's gentle and floral aroma has a calming effect on the nervous system, making it a popular choice for promoting tranquility. Inhaling the scent of chamomile oil through diffusion or direct inhalation can ease tension and soothe the mind. A few drops of diluted chamomile oil applied to the wrists or behind the ears offer a portable and comforting solution for on-the-go stress relief. Additionally, chamomile oil can be added to massage blends or incorporated into nighttime rituals to support restful sleep.

Frankincense essential oil, derived from the resin of the Boswellia sacra tree, has been revered for its grounding and centering effects. Frankincense contains compounds known as boswellic acids, which have been studied for their potential to reduce stress and anxiety. Diffusing frankincense oil or inhaling its aroma directly can create a meditative atmosphere, promoting inner peace and tranquility. Incorporating frankincense oil into mindfulness practices, such as meditation or deep breathing exercises, enhances the overall experience and relieves stress.

Bergamot essential oil, extracted from the peel of the bergamot orange, combines citrusy brightness with calming properties. Rich in compounds like limonene, bergamot oil has uplifting and stress-relieving effects. Diffusing bergamot oil in the home or workplace can create a cheerful environment, helping to counteract feelings of stress. A few drops of diluted bergamot oil applied to the wrists or added to a warm compress provide a soothing and aromatic solution for stress relief. It is important to note that bergamot oil is phototoxic, so caution should be exercised when applying it to the skin before exposure to the sun.

Ylang-ylang essential oil, derived from the flowers of the Cananga odorata tree, is celebrated for its sweet and exotic fragrance. Ylang-ylang oil has soothing properties that can help reduce stress and promote relaxation. Inhaling the floral aroma of ylang-ylang oil through diffusion or direct inhalation can calm the nervous system. Adding a few drops of ylang-ylang oil to a carrier oil for massage or incorporating it into a warm bath provides a luxurious and indulgent way to unwind and release tension.

Clary sage essential oil, obtained from the Salvia sclarea plant, is known for its stress-relieving and mood-enhancing properties. Clary sage oil's musky and herbal aroma has a calming influence on the mind and emotions. Diffusing clary sage oil or inhaling its scent directly can promote a sense of tranquility and emotional balance. A diluted clary sage oil blend applied to the wrists, neck, or temples provides a convenient and portable method for on-the-go stress relief. Clary sage oil mainly benefits women experiencing hormonal fluctuations and stress-related symptoms.

Vetiver essential oil, extracted from the roots of the Vetiveria zizanioides plant, offers grounding and stabilizing effects that make it valuable for stress relief. The earthy and woody aroma of vetiver oil has a calming influence on the mind, helping to reduce anxiety and tension. Diffusing vetiver oil in the evening or inhaling its scent directly before bedtime can contribute to a restful and stress-free sleep. Adding a few drops of vetiver oil to a carrier oil for massage or incorporating it into a relaxation blend enhances its stress-relieving benefits.

The application of essential oils for stress relief and relaxation involves various methods, allowing individuals to choose the approach that best suits their preferences and needs. Diffusion is a popular and effective way to enjoy the aromatic benefits of essential oils throughout the day. Using an ultrasonic diffuser or a simple aromatherapy diffuser allows individuals to disperse the calming scents into the air, creating a tranquil and stress-free environment in their living or working spaces.

Inhalation directly from the bottle or via a personal inhaler offers a quick and portable method for accessing the stress-relieving properties of essential oils. This approach is beneficial during heightened stress or when a calming influence is needed. Inhaling the soothing vapors of selected oils, such as lavender, chamomile, or frankincense, can help ease tension and promote relaxation.

When properly diluted with a carrier oil, the topical application of essential oils allows individuals to experience the stress-relieving effects directly on their skin. Creating a diluted blend and applying it to pulse points, such as the wrists, neck, or temples, enables the absorption of the bioactive compounds. This method effectively sustains a subtle and continuous release of the oils' calming properties throughout the day.

Massage, incorporating stress-relieving essential oils into a carrier oil, offers a dual benefit by combining the therapeutic effects of touch with the aromatic and bioactive properties. A gentle massage using a blend of stress-relieving oils promotes relaxation and contributes to overall emotional well-being. The rhythmic application of the mix allows for enhanced absorption and provides a holistic approach to stress relief.

Baths infused with essential oils provide a luxurious and immersive experience for stress relief and relaxation. Adding a few drops of stress-relieving oils to a warm bath allows the aromatic molecules to be inhaled while the skin absorbs the beneficial compounds. This method is especially effective for addressing overall tension and promoting a sense of calm. Incorporating Epsom salts into the bath can further enhance the therapeutic effects.

Creating personalized blends for stress relief and relaxation allows individuals to tailor their approach to specific needs and preferences. A calming blend for evening relaxation may include lavender, clary sage, and vetiver essential oils combined with a carrier oil for topical application or added to a diffuser for inhalation. Experimenting with basic oil combinations empowers individuals to discover their preferred blends for various stressors and relaxation needs.

In conclusion, essential oils offer a natural and aromatic pathway to stress relief and relaxation. Their calming and soothing properties provide a gentle alternative to synthetic methods, allowing individuals to create moments of tranquility in their daily lives. Whether inhaled through diffusion, applied topically, or incorporated into personalized blends, essential oils provide a versatile and enjoyable means of fostering relaxation and emotional well-being. As with any wellness practice, it is crucial to prioritize safety, proper dilution, and individual considerations. Integrating essential oils into daily routines empowers individuals to tap into the calming and balancing potential of nature's botanical extracts, promoting a holistic and sustainable approach to stress management.

Mood Enhancement

The influence of scents on human emotions and moods has been recognized for centuries, and essential oils derived from aromatic plants have gained popularity for their ability to evoke specific emotional responses. The aromatic compounds in essential oils interact with the olfactory system, influencing the limbic system in the brain, which is closely associated with emotions, memories, and mood regulation. This makes essential oils a natural and powerful tool for enhancing mood and promoting emotional well-being.

Citrus essential oils, including bergamot, lemon, orange, and grapefruit, are renowned for their uplifting and refreshing qualities. The bright and citrusy aromas of these oils stimulate the senses, making them valuable for mood enhancement. Bergamot essential oil, in particular, contains compounds like limonene that contribute to its mood-balancing effects. Diffusing citrus oils in the home or workplace creates an energetic and positive ambiance, helping to counteract feelings of stress and low mood. Inhaling the vibrant scents of citrus oils directly from the bottle or through diffusion provides a quick and effective way to lift spirits and enhance mood.

With its versatile and calming properties, the lavender essential oil is a staple in mood enhancement practices. The soothing aroma of lavender has been associated with relaxation and stress reduction. Inhaling the scent of lavender oil through diffusion or direct inhalation can induce a sense of tranquility and emotional balance. Adding a few drops of lavender oil to a warm bath or applying a diluted solution to pulse points provides a gentle and comforting way to enhance mood. Lavender's ability to promote relaxation makes it a valuable ally in creating a serene atmosphere that supports emotional well-being.

Peppermint essential oil, known for its invigorating and minty scent, offers a refreshing approach to mood enhancement. The active compound menthol in peppermint oil has stimulating mental effects and can help alleviate fatigue. Inhaling the refreshing aroma of peppermint oil through diffusion or direct inhalation provides a quick and revitalizing pick-me-up. Additionally, a diluted solution of peppermint oil applied to the temples or wrists can increase alertness and mood elevation. Peppermint oil's ability to clear the mind makes it popular for enhancing focus and concentration.

Ylang-ylang essential oil, derived from the flowers of the Cananga odorata tree, is prized for its sweet and exotic fragrance with mood-enhancing properties. Ylang-ylang oil has a calming effect on the nervous system and reduces feelings of stress and anxiety. Inhaling the floral aroma of ylang-ylang oil through diffusion or direct inhalation can uplift the spirits and promote a positive mood. Adding a few drops of ylang-ylang oil to a carrier oil for massage or incorporating it into a relaxation blend offers a luxurious and indulgent way to enhance emotional well-being.

Frankincense essential oil, obtained from the resin of the Boswellia sacra tree, is revered for its grounding and centering effects on both the mind and emotions. Frankincense oil's resinous and woody aroma has been associated with spiritual practices and emotional balance. Diffusing frankincense oil or inhaling its scent directly can create a meditative atmosphere, promoting inner peace and uplifting mood. Incorporating frankincense oil into mindfulness or meditation routines enhances the overall experience and improves emotional well-being.

With its rich and intoxicating floral scent, Jasmine essential oil is celebrated for its mood-enhancing and aphrodisiac properties. Jasmine oil has traditionally been used to uplift spirits and evoke joy. Inhaling the sweet and heady aroma of jasmine oil through diffusion or direct inhalation can positively impact mood and emotions. Adding a few drops of jasmine oil to a carrier oil for massage or incorporating it into a personal fragrance allows individuals to experience the mood-enhancing benefits of this luxurious and exotic oil.

Sandalwood essential oil, extracted from the heartwood of sandalwood trees, offers a warm and woody aroma that promotes relaxation and emotional balance. Sandalwood oil has grounding properties that can help calm the mind and reduce feelings of stress. Diffusing sandalwood oil or inhaling its scent directly provides a soothing and meditative experience, contributing to overall well-being. Incorporating sandalwood oil into relaxation rituals or diffusing it in the evening supports a serene and harmonious mood.

Bergamot essential oil, derived from the peel of the bergamot orange, combines citrusy brightness with mood-balancing properties. Bergamot oil contains compounds like limonene and linalool, contributing to its uplifting effects. Diffusing bergamot oil in the home or workplace can create a cheerful environment, helping alleviate anxiety and promote a balanced mood. A few drops of diluted bergamot oil applied to pulse points or added to a personal inhaler provide a convenient and portable solution for mood enhancement.

The application of essential oils for mood enhancement involves various methods, allowing individuals to choose the approach that best suits their preferences and needs. Diffusion is a popular and effective way to enjoy the aromatic benefits of essential oils throughout the day. An ultrasonic or simple aromatherapy diffuser allows individuals to disperse mood-enhancing scents into the air, creating a positive and uplifting atmosphere in their living or working spaces.

Inhalation directly from the bottle or via a personal inhaler offers a quick and portable method for accessing the mood-enhancing properties of essential oils. This approach is beneficial during moments of low energy or when a positive mood boost is needed. Inhaling the delightful scents of selected oils, such as citrus, lavender, or jasmine, can help shift emotional states and create a more positive outlook.

When properly diluted with a carrier oil, the topical application of essential oils allows individuals to experience mood-enhancing effects directly on their skin. Creating a diluted blend and applying it to pulse points, such as the wrists, neck, or temples, enables the absorption of the bioactive compounds. This method effectively sustains a subtle and continuous release of the oils' mood-enhancing properties throughout the day.

Creating personalized blends for mood enhancement allows individuals to tailor their approach to specific needs and preferences. A bright and uplifting blend for morning use may include citrus oils like bergamot, lemon, and orange. Diffusing this blend in the morning or applying it topically can provide a natural and positive start to the day. For relaxation in the evening, a mix of lavender, frankincense, and ylang-ylang can be diffused or applied, creating a serene and mood-balancing atmosphere.

In conclusion, essential oils offer a natural and aromatic avenue for mood enhancement. Their ability to influence emotions and create positive shifts in mood makes them valuable tools for supporting emotional well-being. Whether inhaled through diffusion, applied topically, or incorporated into personalized blends, essential oils provide a versatile and enjoyable means of fostering a positive and balanced emotional state. As with any wellness practice, it is crucial to prioritize safety, proper dilution, and individual considerations. Integrating essential oils into daily routines empowers individuals to tap into the mood-enhancing potential of nature's botanical extracts, promoting a holistic and sustainable approach to emotional well-being.

Sleep Support with Essential Oils

Quality sleep is a cornerstone of overall well-being, impacting physical health, mental clarity, and emotional resilience. Essential oils derived from aromatic plants have gained recognition for their ability to promote relaxation and create a conducive environment for restful sleep. The aromatic compounds in essential oils interact with the olfactory system, influencing the brain's limbic system, which regulates emotions, including stress and relaxation responses. Incorporating essential oils into a bedtime routine offers a natural and aromatic approach to sleep support, helping individuals unwind, alleviate stress, and enjoy a more restful night.

Lavender essential oil is a well-known and widely used oil for sleep support. Renowned for its calming and soothing properties, lavender has a long history of promoting relaxation and reducing anxiety. Inhaling lavender oil's gentle and floral aroma before bedtime, either through diffusion or direct inhalation, signals the nervous system to unwind, creating a tranquil atmosphere conducive to sleep. Additionally, incorporating a few drops of diluted lavender oil into a bedtime massage or a warm bath enhances the overall relaxation experience, contributing to a more restful night's sleep.

Chamomile essential oil, particularly the Roman chamomile variety, is another valuable oil for sleep support. Chamomile's gentle and herbaceous aroma has soothing properties that help calm the mind and induce relaxation. Inhaling the delicate scent of chamomile oil through diffusion or direct inhalation before bedtime promotes a sense of tranquility. A few drops of diluted chamomile oil applied to pulse points or added to a warm compress offer a gentle and aromatic way to ease into a restful sleep. Chamomile oil is particularly beneficial for individuals with insomnia or difficulty falling asleep.

Frankincense essential oil, obtained from the resin of the Boswellia sacra tree, contributes to sleep support with its grounding and centering effects. Frankincense oil has been associated with spiritual practices and relaxation, making it a valuable addition to bedtime routines. Diffusing frankincense oil or inhaling its scent directly before sleep creates a meditative atmosphere, easing the mind into a calm state. Incorporating frankincense oil into relaxation practices, such as deep breathing or meditation, enhances the overall sleep-inducing experience.

Bergamot essential oil, derived from the peel of the bergamot orange, combines citrusy brightness with calming properties, making it an exciting choice for sleep support. Bergamot oil contains compounds like linalool and limonene, contributing to its relaxation effects. Diffusing bergamot oil in the evening or inhaling its aroma directly can create a positive and serene environment, helping to alleviate stress and prepare the mind for sleep. A few drops of diluted bergamot oil applied to pulse points or added to a bedtime blend offer a soothing and aromatic solution for winding down.

Cedarwood essential oil, extracted from the wood of cedar trees, is recognized for its grounding and calming effects on the nervous system. The warm and woody aroma of cedarwood oil promotes a sense of security and relaxation. Diffusing cedarwood oil in the bedroom or inhaling its scent directly before bedtime can contribute to a peaceful and restful sleep environment. Adding a few drops of diluted cedarwood oil to a pillow or incorporating it into a bedtime massage blend provides a comforting and aromatic ritual for sleep support.

Vetiver essential oil, derived from the roots of the Vetiveria zizanioides plant, offers a deep and earthy aroma that promotes relaxation and sleep. Vetiver oil has grounding and soothing properties, making it beneficial for individuals dealing with restlessness or racing thoughts at bedtime. Diffusing vetiver oil in the evening or inhaling its scent directly before sleep can help calm the mind and create a conducive atmosphere for restful slumber. Adding a few drops of diluted vetiver oil to a bedtime blend or applying it to the soles of the feet enhances its sleep-supporting effects.

Lemon balm essential oil, extracted from the leaves of the Melissa officinalis plant, is known for its calming and mild sedative properties. The citrusy and herbaceous aroma of lemon balm oil has a soothing influence on the nervous system. Diffusing lemon balm oil in the bedroom or inhaling its scent directly before bedtime can help promote relaxation and prepare the mind for sleep. Adding a few drops of diluted lemon balm oil to a bedtime massage or a warm bath provides a gentle and aromatic way to support a restful night's sleep.

Applying essential oils for sleep support involves various methods, allowing individuals to choose the approach that best suits their preferences and needs. Diffusion is a popular and effective way to enjoy the aromatic benefits of essential oils throughout the night. Using an ultrasonic diffuser or a simple aromatherapy diffuser allows individuals to disperse the sleep-inducing scents into the air, creating a calming and relaxing atmosphere in their bedroom.

Inhalation directly from the bottle or via a personal inhaler offers a quick and portable method for accessing the sleep-supporting properties of essential oils. This approach benefits individuals who may experience difficulty falling asleep or need support during travel. Inhaling the soothing vapors of selected oils, such as lavender, chamomile, or cedarwood, can help signal the body and mind that it's time to unwind and prepare for sleep.

When properly diluted with a carrier oil, the topical application of essential oils allows individuals to experience the sleep-inducing effects directly on their skin. Creating a diluted blend and applying it to pulse points, such as the wrists, neck, or temples, enables the absorption of the bioactive compounds. This method effectively sustains a subtle and continuous release of the oils' sleep-supporting properties throughout the night. A bedtime massage using a sleep-inducing blend enhances relaxation and provides a more restful sleep.

Baths infused with essential oils provide a luxurious and immersive sleep-support experience. Adding a few drops of sleep-inducing oils to a warm bath allows the aromatic molecules to be inhaled while the skin absorbs the beneficial compounds. This method is particularly effective for individuals dealing with stress or tension that may interfere with sleep. Incorporating Epsom salts into the bath can further enhance the relaxation and sleep-inducing effects.

Creating personalized blends for sleep support allows individuals to tailor their approach to specific needs and preferences. A calming bedtime blend may include lavender, chamomile, and frankincense essential oils combined with a carrier oil for topical application or added to a diffuser for inhalation. Experimenting with basic oil combinations empowers individuals to discover their preferred blends for a restful night's sleep.

In conclusion, essential oils offer a natural and aromatic sleep-support pathway. Their ability to influence the nervous system, induce relaxation, and create a calming environment makes them valuable tools for promoting restful sleep. Whether inhaled through diffusion, applied topically, or incorporated into personalized blends, essential oils provide a versatile and enjoyable means of enhancing sleep quality. As with any wellness practice, it is crucial to prioritize safety, proper dilution, and individual considerations. Integrating essential oils into bedtime routines empowers individuals to tap into the sleep-inducing potential of nature's botanical extracts, fostering a holistic and sustainable approach to achieving restful and rejuvenating sleep.

CHAPTER VII
Integrating Essential Oils into Daily Routines

Creating a Morning Ritual

Creating a morning ritual infused with essential oils' aromatic and refreshing properties can set a positive tone for the day ahead, fostering a sense of intention, balance, and vitality. Essential oils, derived from aromatic plants, contain bioactive compounds that interact with the olfactory system, influencing the limbic system in the brain responsible for emotions, memories, and mood regulation. Incorporating these natural extracts into a morning routine allows one to harness their uplifting and energizing qualities, enhancing overall well-being.

Citrus essential oils, such as bergamot, lemon, orange, and grapefruit, are renowned for their bright and refreshing scents. These oils awaken the senses and provide a burst of energy, making them ideal for a morning ritual. Diffusing citrus oils in the morning creates a vibrant and positive atmosphere, helping to dispel grogginess and elevate mood. Inhaling the refreshing aroma of citrus oils directly from the bottle or through diffusion signals the brain to wake up and embrace the new day. The citrusy notes of these oils add a touch of freshness to the morning routine, creating a sensory experience that encourages alertness and positivity.

Peppermint essential oil is a dynamic addition to a morning ritual with its refreshing and minty aroma. The active compound menthol in peppermint oil stimulates the mind and can help increase alertness. Inhaling the revitalizing scent of peppermint oil through diffusion or direct inhalation provides a quick and refreshing pick-me-up. Adding a few drops of diluted peppermint oil to a morning shower gel or applying it to the back of the neck creates a cooling sensation, contributing to a sense of wakefulness and mental clarity. Peppermint oil's ability to clear the mind makes it a valuable ally for starting the day with focus and energy.

Eucalyptus essential oil, known for its refreshing and respiratory benefits, adds fresh air to a morning ritual. The crisp and camphorous aroma of eucalyptus oil can help clear nasal passages and promote a sense of vitality. Diffusing eucalyptus oil in the morning or inhaling its scent directly can be especially beneficial during seasonal changes or when looking to invigorate the respiratory system. The aromatic profile of eucalyptus oil adds a revitalizing element to the morning routine, contributing to a feeling of rejuvenation and readiness for the day ahead.

Lemon balm essential oil, extracted from the leaves of the Melissa officinalis plant, offers a calming and citrusy aroma that promotes focus and mental clarity. Inhaling the refreshing scent of lemon balm oil through diffusion or direct inhalation in the morning can help create a centered and balanced mindset. Adding a few drops of diluted lemon balm oil to a diffuser blend or applying it to pulse points provides a gentle and aromatic way to enhance concentration and promote a positive outlook. Lemon balm oil's ability to soothe the mind makes it a valuable asset for individuals seeking a mindful and intentional start to their day.

Rosemary essential oil, derived from the aromatic herb Rosmarinus officinalis, is known for its cognitive-enhancing properties. The refreshing and herbaceous aroma of rosemary oil has been associated with improved focus, memory, and mental alertness. Diffusing rosemary oil in the morning or inhaling its scent directly can stimulate the mind and promote a sense of wakefulness. Incorporating rosemary oil into a morning blend for massage or applying it to pulse points contributes to cognitive support, making it an excellent choice for individuals looking to kickstart their day with mental clarity and sharpness.

Creating a morning ritual with essential oils involves various methods, allowing individuals to tailor their approach to specific needs and preferences. Diffusion is a popular and effective way to enjoy the aromatic benefits of essential oils throughout the morning. An ultrasonic or simple aromatherapy diffuser allows individuals to disperse the invigorating scents into the air, creating an energizing and positive atmosphere in their living or working spaces.

Inhalation directly from the bottle or via a personal inhaler offers a quick and portable method for accessing the uplifting properties of essential oils. This approach benefits individuals needing a natural energy boost during the morning commute or transitioning from home to work. Inhaling the revitalizing scents of selected oils, such as citrus, peppermint, or rosemary, can help set a positive and focused tone for the day.

When properly diluted with a carrier oil, the topical application of essential oils allows individuals to experience the invigorating effects directly on their skin. Creating a diluted blend and applying it to pulse points, such as the wrists, neck, or temples, enables the absorption of the bioactive compounds. This method effectively sustains a subtle and continuous release of the oils' energizing properties throughout the morning. A morning massage using a blend of uplifting oils provides a sensory and revitalizing experience.

Incorporating essential oils into morning skincare or grooming routines offers a multi-sensory approach to starting the day. Adding a few drops of a refreshing oil, such as citrus or peppermint, to a facial cleanser, moisturizer, or shaving cream can provide a vital and aromatic element to the morning routine. The sensory experience of the oils enhances the overall ritual, creating a positive and uplifting environment for the day ahead.

Mindful practices, such as deep breathing or meditation, can be enhanced by the aromatic support of essential oils. Diffusing calming oils like lavender or frankincense during a morning meditation session creates a serene and focused atmosphere. Inhaling the soothing scents of these oils allows individuals to center themselves and set positive intentions for the day. Incorporating mindfulness into a morning ritual with essential oils provides a holistic approach to well-being, addressing mental and emotional aspects.

In conclusion, incorporating essential oils into a morning ritual offers a natural and aromatic approach to starting the day with intention and vitality. The invigorating scents of citrus, peppermint, eucalyptus, lemon balm, and rosemary oils contribute to a positive and energized mindset. Whether diffused, inhaled, applied topically, or integrated into mindfulness practices, essential oils provide a versatile and enjoyable means of enhancing the morning routine. As with any wellness practice, it is crucial to prioritize safety, proper dilution, and individual considerations. Integrating essential oils into morning rituals empowers individuals to tap into the uplifting and energizing potential of nature's botanical extracts, fostering a holistic and sustainable approach to well-being.

Essential Oils in Self-Care Practices

In modern self-care practices, essential oils have emerged as powerful and versatile allies, contributing to physical, emotional, and mental well-being. Derived from aromatic plants, these concentrated extracts contain bioactive compounds that interact with the body and mind, offering a natural and holistic approach to self-care. Incorporating essential oils into self-care routines enhances the overall experience, providing individuals with a sensory and therapeutic pathway to relaxation, rejuvenation, and balance.

One of the primary ways essential oils contribute to self-care is through their ability to promote relaxation and alleviate stress. In today's fast-paced and demanding world, stress has become ubiquitous in daily life, impacting both physical and mental health. Essential oils such as lavender, chamomile, and frankincense are renowned for their calming properties. Inhaling the soothing aroma of lavender oil, either through diffusion or direct inhalation, signals the brain to induce relaxation, helping to ease tension and stress. Similarly, chamomile essential oil, with its gentle and herbaceous scent, has a tranquilizing effect on the nervous system, making it an ideal companion for moments of self-care. Frankincense essential oil, often associated with spiritual practices, has grounding properties that help individuals find a sense of balance and calm amidst the chaos of daily life.

In addition to stress relief, essential oils support emotional well-being. The aromatic compounds in oils like bergamot, ylang-ylang, and rose can uplift the spirits and promote a positive mindset. Bergamot essential oil, derived from the peel of the bergamot orange, combines citrusy brightness with mood-balancing properties. Diffusing bergamot oil in the home or workplace can create a cheerful environment, helping to alleviate anxiety and promote emotional balance. Ylang-ylang essential oil, celebrated for its sweet and exotic fragrance, has soothing properties that can reduce stress and promote relaxation, contributing to emotional well-being. Rose essential oil, derived from the petals of the rose flower, is associated with feelings of love and comfort. Inhaling the floral aroma of rose oil can have a soothing effect on emotions, making it a valuable addition to self-care practices focused on nurturing the spirit.

Integrating essential oils into skincare routines enhances the sensory experience of self-care, providing physical and emotional benefits. Oils such as tea tree, lavender, and chamomile are well-suited for skincare, offering properties that support healthy skin and contribute to a luxurious and nurturing self-care ritual. Tea tree essential oil, known for its antimicrobial properties, can be added to skincare formulations to address blemishes and promote clear skin. With its soothing and anti-inflammatory properties, the lavender essential oil is gentle on the skin and can be incorporated into skincare products or applied topically to calm irritated skin. Chamomile essential oil, particularly the Roman chamomile variety, is celebrated for its anti-inflammatory and calming effects, making it an excellent choice for sensitive skin. Incorporating these oils into skincare practices transforms routine tasks into moments of self-indulgence, fostering a deeper connection with oneself and promoting a radiant complexion.

Aromatherapy, the practice of using essential oils for therapeutic purposes, is a cornerstone of self-care that engages the sense of smell to influence emotions and promote well-being. Diffusing essential oils, such as eucalyptus, peppermint, or lemon, creates an aromatic ambiance that enhances the overall self-care experience. With its refreshing and respiratory benefits, Eucalyptus essential oil can be diffused to promote clear breathing and a sense of vitality. Peppermint essential oil, known for its stimulating and energizing properties, uplifts the mood and contributes to mental clarity when diffused. With its bright and citrusy aroma, Lemon essential oil creates a positive and uplifting atmosphere, making it an excellent choice for enhancing self-care rituals.

Massage, combined with the therapeutic benefits of essential oils, becomes a holistic self-care practice that addresses physical and emotional well-being. Oils such as lavender, chamomile, and eucalyptus are popular for massage blends, offering relaxation, calming effects, and respiratory support. Lavender essential oil, diluted with a carrier oil, can be applied through gentle massage to promote relaxation and release muscle tension. With its anti-inflammatory properties, chamomile essential oil contributes to a soothing and comforting massage experience. When blended with a carrier oil, Eucalyptus essential oil provides a cooling and refreshing sensation, making it suitable for massage practices focused on revitalization and tension relief. The combination of touch and aroma in a massage with essential oils enhances the self-care journey, fostering a sense of connection and rejuvenation.

Essential oils also find their place in mindfulness and meditation, enriching the self-care experience with a deeper connection to the present moment. Oils such as frankincense, sandalwood, and cedarwood are revered for their grounding and centering effects, making them valuable companions for contemplative practices. Frankincense essential oil, with its resinous and woody aroma, has been used in spiritual rituals for centuries. Inhaling the scent of frankincense oil during meditation creates a meditative atmosphere, promoting inner peace and tranquility. Sandalwood essential oil, extracted from the heartwood of sandalwood trees, has a warm and woody aroma that encourages focus and mental clarity during mindfulness practices. With its grounding properties, Cedarwood essential oil supports a centered and balanced state of mind, making it an excellent choice for meditation. Incorporating essential oils into mindfulness elevates the sensory experience, facilitating a deeper connection with oneself and the surrounding environment.

In conclusion, essential oils are valuable companions in self-care practices, enhancing physical, emotional, and mental well-being. From stress relief and emotional balance to skincare and aromatherapy, these aromatic extracts contribute to a holistic and sensory approach to self-care. Whether diffused, applied topically, or incorporated into massage and mindfulness practices, essential oils offer a versatile and enjoyable means of nurturing oneself. As with any wellness practice, it is crucial to prioritize safety, proper dilution, and individual considerations. Integrating essential oils into self-care routines empowers individuals to tap into the therapeutic potential of nature's botanical extracts, fostering a holistic and sustainable approach to well-being.

Enhancing Your Evening Routine

As the day winds down and the demands of daily life ease, the evening becomes an opportune time to engage in self-care practices that promote relaxation, balance, and a restful transition into the night. Essential oils, derived from aromatic plants, play a significant role in enhancing the evening routine, offering a natural and therapeutic approach to unwinding the body and the mind. Whether through diffusion, topical application, or incorporation into evening rituals such as baths and bedtime routines, essential oils provide a serene and rejuvenating experience that prepares individuals for a restful night's sleep.

Lavender essential oil, revered for its calming and soothing properties, enhances the evening routine. The gentle and floral aroma of lavender has a long-standing reputation for promoting relaxation and reducing anxiety. Diffusing lavender oil in the evening creates a tranquil atmosphere, signaling the nervous system to unwind and prepare for sleep. Inhaling the soothing scent of lavender oil directly or incorporating a few drops into a bedtime bath provides a sensory and calming experience, making it an essential companion for those seeking to transition seamlessly from the hustle of the day to the tranquility of the evening.

Chamomile essential oil, particularly the Roman chamomile variety, is another valuable addition to the evening routine. Known for its gentle and herbaceous aroma, chamomile oil has soothing properties that can help induce relaxation and alleviate stress. Diffusing chamomile oil in the evening or inhaling its scent directly before bedtime promotes a sense of tranquility. Adding a few drops of diluted chamomile oil to a warm compress or incorporating it into a massage blend contributes to a soothing and aromatic prelude to sleep. Chamomile oil's ability to calm the nervous system makes it an excellent choice for individuals looking to unwind and release tension in the evening.

Frankincense essential oil, obtained from the resin of the Boswellia sacra tree, contributes to the evening routine with its grounding and centering effects. Frankincense oil's resinous and woody aroma has been associated with spiritual practices and emotional balance. Diffusing frankincense oil in the evening or inhaling its scent directly creates a meditative atmosphere, fostering a sense of inner peace and tranquility. Incorporating frankincense oil into mindfulness or relaxation practices, such as deep breathing exercises, enhances the overall evening experience, preparing the mind for a restful night's sleep.

Bergamot essential oil, derived from the peel of the bergamot orange, combines citrusy brightness with mood-balancing properties, making it a delightful addition to the evening routine. Bergamot oil contains compounds like limonene and linalool, contributing to its uplifting effects. Diffusing bergamot oil in the evening can create a cheerful environment, helping to alleviate stress and promote emotional balance. A few drops of diluted bergamot oil applied to pulse points or incorporated into a relaxation blend offers a soothing and aromatic solution for winding down after a busy day.

Cedarwood essential oil, extracted from the wood of cedar trees, is recognized for its grounding and calming effects on the nervous system. The warm and woody aroma of cedarwood oil contributes to a serene atmosphere in the evening. Diffusing cedarwood oil before bedtime or inhaling its scent directly promotes relaxation and mental tranquility. Adding a few drops of diluted cedarwood oil to a nighttime massage blend or incorporating it into a bedtime routine provides a comforting and aromatic ritual that signals the body and mind to prepare for sleep. Cedarwood oil's ability to induce a sense of security and calmness makes it a valuable asset in creating an evening sanctuary.

Ylang-ylang essential oil, derived from the flowers of the Cananga odorata tree, offers a sweet and exotic fragrance with mood-enhancing properties. In the evening, ylang-ylang oil contributes to a relaxing and indulgent experience. Diffusing ylang-ylang oil before bedtime or inhaling its scent directly promotes a positive and serene mood. Adding a few drops of diluted ylang-ylang oil to a warm bath or incorporating it into a bedtime massage blend enhances the evening routine, creating a luxurious and aromatic atmosphere that supports emotional well-being and relaxation.

Creating an evening routine with essential oils involves various methods, allowing individuals to tailor their approach to specific needs and preferences. Diffusion remains a popular and effective way to enjoy the aromatic benefits of essential oils during the evening. An ultrasonic or simple aromatherapy diffuser allows individuals to disperse calming scents into the air, creating a peaceful and relaxing atmosphere in their living or sleeping spaces.

Inhalation directly from the bottle or via a personal inhaler offers a quick and portable method for accessing the calming properties of essential oils. This approach benefits individuals needing support in unwinding during travel or when transitioning from work to home. Inhaling the soothing scents of selected oils, such as lavender, chamomile, or ylang-ylang, can help create a sense of serenity and relaxation in the evening.

When properly diluted with a carrier oil, the topical application of essential oils allows individuals to experience the calming effects directly on their skin. Creating a diluted blend and applying it to pulse points, such as the wrists, neck, or temples, enables the absorption of the bioactive compounds. This method effectively sustains a subtle and continuous release of the oils' calming properties throughout the evening. A gentle massage using an evening blend contributes to relaxation and prepares the body for restful sleep.

Incorporating essential oils into an evening skincare routine enhances the sensory experience and provides additional benefits for skin health. Adding a few drops of calming oils, such as lavender or chamomile, to a nighttime moisturizer or facial oil creates a luxurious and aromatic treatment for the skin. The soothing properties of these oils contribute to a relaxing skincare ritual, promoting both physical and emotional well-being.

Baths infused with essential oils offer a luxurious and immersive experience for the evening routine. Adding a few drops of calming oils to a warm bath allows the aromatic molecules to be inhaled while the skin absorbs the beneficial compounds. This method is particularly effective for individuals dealing with stress or tension that may interfere with a restful night's sleep. Incorporating Epsom salts into the bath enhances the relaxation and soothing effects, creating a therapeutic and indulgent evening ritual.

Mindful practices, such as meditation or gentle stretching, can be enhanced by the aromatic support of essential oils. Diffusing oils like frankincense or cedarwood during an evening meditation session creates a serene and focused atmosphere. Inhaling the grounding scents of these oils allows individuals to center themselves and release the day's tensions. Incorporating mindfulness into an evening routine with essential oils provides a holistic approach to relaxation, addressing both physical and mental aspects.

In conclusion, essential oils offer a natural and aromatic pathway to enhancing the evening routine. The calming and soothing properties of lavender, chamomile, frankincense, bergamot, cedarwood, and ylang-ylang contribute to a tranquil and restful atmosphere. Whether diffused, inhaled, applied topically, or incorporated into baths and skincare rituals, essential oils provide a versatile and enjoyable means of creating a serene and rejuvenating evening experience. As with any wellness practice, it is crucial to prioritize safety, proper dilution, and individual considerations. Integrating essential oils into the evening routine empowers individuals to tap into the therapeutic potential of nature's botanical extracts, fostering a holistic and sustainable approach to relaxation and well-being.

CHAPTER VIII
Exploring Advanced Blending Techniques

Understanding Notes in Essential Oils

Understanding the intricate world of essential oils involves delving into the concept of notes, a fundamental aspect that defines the aromatic profile, longevity, and overall composition of these precious extracts. In perfumery and aromatherapy, the term "notes" refers to the classification of aromatic components based on their evaporation rates. Essential oils comprise a complex mixture of volatile compounds with unique scents, therapeutic properties, and evaporation rates. By categorizing these compounds into top, middle, and base notes, practitioners and enthusiasts gain insights into how oils interact, blend, and contribute to the overall olfactory experience.

Starting with the top notes are the initial scents that greet the senses when an essential oil is first encountered. Top notes are characterized by their light, fresh, and often citrusy aromas. They are the most volatile components, evaporating quickly and providing the first impression of a blend. Examples of top-note essential oils include citruses like lemon, orange, and bergamot and herbal oils such as peppermint and eucalyptus. The refreshing and uplifting qualities of top notes make them ideal for creating a sense of alertness and freshness, making them well-suited for daytime or energizing blends.

Moving on to the middle notes, also known as heart notes, these scents emerge once the top notes have dissipated. Middle notes contribute to the body and fullness of an essential oil blend, creating a harmonious transition between the initial burst of aroma and the more enduring base notes. Middle notes are often floral, herbal, or spicy, adding complexity to the fragrance. Familiar middle note essential oils include lavender, rosemary, chamomile, and geranium. These oils balance a blend, bridging the fleeting top notes and the deeper, lingering base notes.

Base notes form the foundation of an essential oil blend, offering richness, depth, and longevity. These notes are characterized by their heavy, earthy, and grounding aromas. Base notes evaporate slowly, lingering on the skin and in the air for an extended period. Essential oils in this category include woody scents like cedarwood and sandalwood, resinous oils like frankincense and myrrh, and rich and balsamic aromas such as vanilla and patchouli. Base notes contribute to the overall longevity of a blend and provide a sense of warmth, stability, and depth, making them essential for creating well-rounded and enduring fragrances.

Understanding the interplay of top, middle, and base notes is crucial for crafting balanced and harmonious essential oil blends. A well-structured blend includes a thoughtful combination of notes to create a dynamic and evolving olfactory experience. For example, a refreshing and energizing blend might start with top notes like citrus oils for a refreshing burst, followed by middle notes like lavender or peppermint to add complexity, and anchored by base notes like cedarwood or patchouli for a lasting and comforting finish.

Furthermore, the concept of notes extends beyond individual oils to the overall composition of a blend. Essential oil practitioners often refer to the "note pyramid" or "fragrance pyramid" to visualize the arrangement of notes in a particular blend. The pyramid concept reflects the hierarchy of evaporation rates, with top notes at the top, then middle notes in the middle, and base notes at the base. This visual representation aids in the strategic layering of scents, ensuring a well-balanced and cohesive aromatic experience.

Beyond their role in perfumery, the understanding of notes in essential oils is integral to the practice of aromatherapy. Different notes carry distinct therapeutic properties, and their evaporation rates influence the duration and intensity of these effects. For example, top notes with quick evaporation are often chosen for their uplifting and invigorating qualities, making them suitable for addressing momentary emotional states like stress or fatigue. Middle notes contribute to emotional balance and can have a calming or uplifting effect over an extended period, while base notes provide a foundation for relaxation and grounding, supporting emotional well-being over an extended duration.

Blending essential oils requires a nuanced understanding of each oil's note, allowing practitioners to create harmonious and effective combinations tailored to specific needs. Whether aiming for a calming blend to promote relaxation or an energizing blend to enhance focus, notes' thoughtful selection and layering play a pivotal role in achieving the desired aromatic and therapeutic outcomes.

As with any art form, there is an element of subjectivity in the appreciation and composition of essential oil blends. Personal preferences, cultural influences, and individual sensitivities contribute to the diverse world of aromatic experiences. Exploring and experimenting with different notes allows enthusiasts to develop a deeper connection to the nuances of each oil and hone their skills in crafting blends that resonate with their unique preferences.

In conclusion, understanding notes in essential oils is critical in the artistic and therapeutic applications of these aromatic extracts. The classification of top, middle, and base notes provide a framework for comprehending the olfactory journey of a blend, from the initial impression to the lingering aftereffects. This knowledge empowers practitioners and enthusiasts to create blends that delight the senses and offer nuanced and targeted therapeutic benefits. Exploring notes adds depth to the experience of working with essential oils, inviting individuals to embark on a sensory journey as diverse and individualized as the oils themselves.

Crafting Personalized Blends

Crafting personalized blends using essential oils is both an art and a science, allowing individuals to tailor aromatic experiences that align with their unique preferences, needs, and intentions. Essential oils, derived from aromatic plants, are versatile tools that offer a broad spectrum of scents and therapeutic properties. Creating personalized blends involves a thoughtful combination of different oils, each selected for its distinct aroma, note, and potential benefits. Whether aiming to enhance mood, address specific health concerns, or create a signature scent, blending essential oils provides a creative and holistic approach to well-being.

The foundation of crafting personalized blends lies in a fundamental understanding of individual oils, their notes, and the synergy that can be achieved through strategic combinations. Each essential oil carries its character, ranging from the bright and uplifting notes of citrus oils to the grounding and earthy tones of woods and resins. By exploring the aromatic profiles of various oils, individuals can build a palette of scents that resonates with their preferences and objectives.

The first step in crafting a personalized blend is identifying the primary purpose or theme of the blend. Whether seeking relaxation, energy, focus, or a sense of balance, defining the intention behind the mix serves as a guiding principle for selecting the appropriate oils. For instance, if the goal is to create a calming blend for stress relief, oils with soothing properties like lavender, chamomile, and frankincense may be considered. Alternatively, if the aim is to boost energy and concentration, invigorating oils such as peppermint, rosemary, and citrus oils might take center stage.

Understanding the notes of essential oils is crucial in achieving a well-balanced and harmonious blend. The concept of top, middle, and base notes come into play, with each note contributing to the overall olfactory experience and therapeutic effects. Top notes, being the most volatile, provide the initial impression and freshness of the blend. Middle notes contribute body and complexity, while base notes offer depth and longevity. A thoughtful selection of oils from each category ensures the blend unfolds over time, creating a dynamic and evolving aromatic journey.

Experimentation is a crucial aspect of crafting personalized blends. It involves exploring different combinations of oils, adjusting ratios, and fine-tuning the blend to achieve the desired effect. Creating small test batches allows individuals to experience the mix in different contexts and observe how the oils interact over time. The process of experimentation encourages a playful and intuitive approach, inviting individuals to trust their senses and instincts in the quest for the perfect blend.

In addition to the olfactory aspect, considering each oil's therapeutic properties enhances the blend's overall effectiveness. Essential oils offer a range of benefits, including anti-inflammatory, antibacterial, calming, and uplifting properties. Integrating oils with complementary therapeutic effects ensures that the blend smells pleasing and addresses specific well-being goals. For example, blending lavender and eucalyptus can create a synergy that promotes relaxation and respiratory support.

The art of crafting personalized blends extends beyond standalone aromas to creating thematic blends that evoke specific moods or experiences. Seasonal blends, for instance, allow individuals to connect with the changing seasons and create a sensory experience that aligns with nature. A winter blend might include warm and comforting oils like cinnamon and clove, while a summer blend could feature citrus and floral notes for a refreshing and uplifting atmosphere. By infusing blends with intention and thematic elements, individuals can use aromatherapy to enhance their connection to the environment and create a holistic sense of well-being.

Personalized blends also apply in daily life, from skincare to home environments. Creating a custom skincare blend involves selecting oils that address specific skin concerns while providing a pleasant aroma. For example, blending tea tree oil with lavender and chamomile can create a soothing and antibacterial blend for skincare. Similarly, crafting a room spray or diffuser blend allows individuals to infuse their living spaces with scents that promote relaxation, focus, or a sense of cleanliness.

Crafting personalized blends fosters a deeper connection with essential oils and an increased awareness of their effects on the body and mind. It encourages individuals to approach well-being holistically, considering both aromatherapy's sensory and therapeutic aspects. As the blend reflects individual preferences and intentions, it transforms into a personal ritual that enhances daily rituals and promotes a sense of self-care.

Furthermore, crafting personalized blends invites a mindful and present approach to well-being. It encourages individuals to be attuned to their senses, observe each oil's subtle nuances, and embrace the creative process of blending. This mindfulness extends beyond the blending session, fostering an ongoing awareness of the aromatic choices made in daily life. Whether diffusing a calming blend before bedtime or applying a focus blend during work hours, the intentional use of personalized blends becomes a conscious act of self-care.

For those new to the world of essential oils, creating personalized blends offers an entry point into the diverse and enriching realm of aromatherapy. Starting with a small collection of oils and experimenting with crucial blends provides a hands-on and accessible introduction to blending. As confidence grows and familiarity with oils deepens, individuals can expand their repertoire, exploring more complex combinations and refining their blending skills.

In conclusion, crafting personalized blends using essential oils is a dynamic and rewarding endeavor that combines artistry with intentionality. It empowers individuals to curate their olfactory experiences, addressing specific well-being goals and infusing daily life with aromas that resonate with their unique preferences. The process of blending invites exploration, experimentation, and a mindful connection to the sensory delights of essential oils. From enhancing mood to promoting relaxation, crafting personalized blends offers a holistic approach to well-being that celebrates the individuality of each person's aromatic journey.

Safety Measures in Blending

Ensuring safety in blending essential oils is paramount, as these potent extracts demand careful consideration and respect for their concentrated nature. While the creative process of crafting personalized blends can be a delightful and therapeutic pursuit, it is crucial to implement strict safety measures to mitigate potential risks and maximize the benefits of aromatherapy. From proper dilution ratios to understanding individual sensitivities, a comprehensive approach to safety protects the user and enhances the overall effectiveness and enjoyment of essential oil blending.

One fundamental safety measure in blending essential oils is mastering the art of dilution. Essential oils are highly concentrated extracts, and their direct application to the skin can lead to adverse reactions, such as irritation or sensitization. Diluting essential oils in a carrier oil, such as jojoba, almond, or coconut oil, not only ensures safer application but also aids in the even distribution of the blend. The recommended dilution ratio varies depending on the specific essential oil, the intended use, and the individual's age and health condition. A general guideline is to use a 2% dilution for adults, translating to approximately 12 drops of essential oil per ounce of carrier oil. The recommended dilution is much lower for children, typically around 0.5% to 1%. This dilution practice strikes a balance between harnessing the therapeutic benefits of essential oils and safeguarding against potential adverse reactions.

Additionally, understanding the concept of phototoxicity is crucial in ensuring safe blending practices. Certain essential oils, particularly citrus oils like bergamot, lemon, and lime, contain compounds that make the skin more sensitive to sunlight. Direct exposure to UV rays after applying phototoxic oils can result in skin irritation, burns, or discoloration. To prevent phototoxic reactions, avoiding applying phototoxic oils to exposed skin before sun exposure is essential. If inclusion in a blend is desired, such oils can be used in the evening or in products that will not be exposed to sunlight, such as nighttime skincare formulations or relaxation blends.

Another vital safety aspect in blending essential oils involves understanding individual sensitivities and potential allergic reactions. While essential oils are generally well-tolerated, some individuals may have sensitivities or allergies to specific oils. Conducting a patch test before widespread application can help identify any adverse reactions. To perform a patch test, dilute the essential oil in a carrier oil and apply a small amount to a discreet skin area, such as the inner forearm. Monitor the area for 24 hours, checking for signs of redness, itching, or irritation. If any adverse reactions occur, avoiding using that particular oil or adjusting the dilution ratio is advisable.

Furthermore, considering age and vulnerability is crucial when blending essential oils, especially when creating blends for children, older people, or individuals with compromised immune systems. Children have more delicate skin and higher absorption rates, making them more susceptible to adverse reactions. It is essential to adhere to age-appropriate dilution ratios and choose oils deemed safe for specific age groups. Similarly, individuals with certain health conditions or medical treatments should exercise caution and consult healthcare professionals before incorporating essential oils into their routines.

Selecting high-quality, pure essential oils from reputable sources is a foundational safety measure in blending. Adulterated or synthetic oils may contain impurities that can pose health risks. Choosing oils from trusted suppliers that provide transparency regarding sourcing, testing, and purity ensures that the oils used in blends are of the highest quality. Additionally, adhering to recommended storage guidelines, such as keeping oils in dark glass bottles away from direct sunlight and extreme temperatures, helps maintain their integrity and potency.

An often-overlooked safety measure involves acknowledging the potential interactions between essential oils and medications. Some essential oils may interfere with certain medicines by enhancing or inhibiting their effects. Individuals on medication must consult with healthcare professionals before incorporating new crucial oils into their routines. This precautionary step helps prevent any unintended interactions that could compromise the effectiveness of drugs or lead to adverse effects.

Beyond physical safety, it is essential to prioritize emotional well-being when blending essential oils. Aromas can evoke powerful emotions and memories, and certain scents may trigger negative responses in some individuals. Personal preferences, cultural sensitivities, and individual associations with specific aromas contribute to a positive and enjoyable blending experience. Ensuring that the chosen scents align with the intended emotional and therapeutic goals promotes a harmonious and supportive aromatic journey.

Implementing safety measures also extends to storing and handling essential oils during the blending process. Essential oils are volatile compounds that can evaporate over time, especially if exposed to air and light. Tightly sealing bottles and storing them in a cool, dark place helps preserve the oils' freshness and potency. When blending, using clean and dry utensils, such as glass droppers or stainless steel spoons, prevents contamination and maintains the purity of the oils. Practicing good hygiene during the blending process, including washing hands and work surfaces, adds an extra layer of safety and ensures the integrity of the final blend.

Moreover, ongoing commitment to education is integral to safe blending practices. The field of aromatherapy is continually evolving, with new research and insights emerging. Staying informed about developments in essential oil safety, applications, and research findings ensures that blending practices align with the latest knowledge. Engaging in courses, workshops, or consulting reputable aromatherapy resources helps build a strong foundation of knowledge and promotes a culture of safety within the aromatherapy community.

In conclusion, safety measures in blending essential oils are essential for maximizing the benefits and minimizing potential risks associated with these potent extracts. From proper dilution and awareness of phototoxicity to understanding individual sensitivities and considering emotional well-being, a holistic approach to safety enhances the overall enjoyment and efficacy of essential oil blending. By prioritizing quality, education, and thoughtful application, individuals can embark on a journey of aromatherapy that is both creative and therapeutic and safe and respectful of the potent nature of essential oils.

CHAPTER IX
Essential Oils for Special Occasions

Aromatherapy for Celebrations

Aromatherapy, with its profound impact on emotions and well-being, emerges as a delightful and meaningful addition to celebrations, offering a sensorial dimension that elevates the festive atmosphere. Whether it's a joyous gathering, a milestone event, or a traditional ceremony, aromatherapy can enhance the overall experience by engaging the olfactory senses, evoking memories, and creating an ambiance that resonates with the essence of the occasion. Using essential oils in aromatherapy for celebrations is a thoughtful and versatile practice that can be incorporated in various ways, from creating signature scents to enhancing relaxation during festivities.

One of the most impactful ways to infuse aromatherapy into celebrations is by crafting signature scents that become synonymous with the event. A personalized blend of essential oils, carefully chosen to reflect the theme or mood of the celebration, can leave a lasting impression on attendees. A blend featuring floral notes like rose, jasmine, and lavender may evoke romance and elegance for a wedding. A festive holiday gathering could be enhanced by blending warm and spicy oils like cinnamon, clove, and orange, creating a cozy and inviting atmosphere. The key is to select oils that resonate with the emotions and themes associated with the celebration, turning the event into a multisensory experience.

Diffusion is a popular method for introducing aromatherapy into celebratory spaces. Using essential oil diffusers or aroma diffusing machines allows the chosen scents to permeate the air, enveloping the venue in a fragrant embrace. Whether it's the entrance of a party, the dining area, or the dance floor, the strategic placement of diffusers ensures a consistent and immersive aromatic experience for all attendees. The gentle diffusion of essential oils contributes to a dynamic atmosphere, subtly evolving as the celebration progresses and adding a layer of sophistication to the sensory landscape.

Aromatherapy can also be seamlessly integrated into celebratory rituals, creating moments of relaxation and connection. For instance, incorporating scented oils into massage stations or event relaxation areas offers attendees a chance to unwind and indulge in a sensory respite. Oils with calming properties, such as lavender or chamomile, can be used in massage blends, creating a serene and rejuvenating experience. This approach not only enhances the overall well-being of attendees but also adds a touch of luxury to the celebration, making it a memorable and holistic experience.

In addition to diffusion and massage, scented candles and incense are timeless elements that bring an element of ritual and elegance to celebrations. Candles infused with essential oils provide ambient lighting and release subtle fragrances as they burn. Whether it's the warm glow of candles on dining tables or the ethereal ambiance created by strategically placed incense, these elements contribute to the overall sensory tapestry of the celebration. The flickering flames and aromatic trails become integral components of the festive environment, enhancing the mood and creating an immersive experience.

Celebratory moments often involve rituals and ceremonies that hold cultural or personal significance. Aromatherapy can be woven into these rituals, adding depth and intentionality. For example, anointing ceremony participants with oils that carry symbolic or meaningful scents can create a profound and memorable experience. Oils with spiritual or ceremonial significance, such as frankincense or myrrh, can be incorporated into these rituals, aligning the aromatic elements with the deeper meaning of the celebration.

Furthermore, aromatherapy for celebrations extends beyond the event itself, as scents uniquely evoke memories. Creating scented keepsakes, such as scented sachets or personalized essential oil blends, allows attendees to carry a piece of the celebration. These tokens become olfactory mementos, triggering memories and emotions whenever the scent is encountered in the future. The power of scent in evoking nostalgia adds a timeless and enduring dimension to the celebration, creating a sensory bridge between past and present.

When planning aromatherapy for celebrations, it is essential to consider the preferences and sensitivities of attendees. Opting for universally appealing scents like citrus or florals ensures a broadly enjoyable experience. Additionally, providing options for personalization, such as allowing attendees to choose scents for their massage oils or offering a variety of diffuser blends, adds an inclusive and participatory element to the aromatic journey.

In conclusion, aromatherapy for celebrations transforms festive occasions into multisensory experiences, infusing events with intentionality, elegance, and emotional resonance. From crafting signature scents to incorporating oils into rituals and providing moments of relaxation, aromatherapy enhances the overall well-being of attendees and creates a lasting impact. Whether it's the warm and inviting glow of scented candles, the immersive diffusion of essential oils, or the creation of scented keepsakes, aromatherapy contributes to cherished memories. As celebrations become opportunities for connection and reflection, the artful use of essential oils adds a layer of sophistication and meaning, elevating the experience of joyous occasions.

Creating a Relaxing Environment for Guests

Creating a relaxing environment for guests through the strategic use of essential oils is a thoughtful and impactful way to enhance their overall experience. The ability of aromas to influence mood and evoke emotions makes them a valuable tool for setting the tone and ambiance of a space. Whether it's a home gathering, a spa day, or a hospitality setting, incorporating essential oils into the environment contributes to a sense of tranquility, comfort, and well-being for guests.

One of the most effective ways to establish a relaxing atmosphere is by using essential oil diffusers. These devices disperse the aromatic molecules of essential oils into the air, creating a subtle and continuous infusion of fragrance throughout the space. Diffusers come in various styles, from ultrasonic to nebulizing, providing flexibility in choosing the most suitable option for the setting. A carefully selected blend of calming essential oils, such as lavender, chamomile, and bergamot, diffused in the environment instantly invites guests into a soothing and inviting ambiance. This approach is efficient in communal areas, such as living rooms or reception areas, where the collective olfactory experience contributes to a shared sense of relaxation.

In addition to diffusers, scented candles infused with essential oils are a classic and elegant way to create a tranquil environment. The warm glow of candlelight combined with the gentle release of fragrant oils adds a sensory layer to the visual and aromatic experience. Candles can be strategically placed where guests gather, such as dining tables or relaxation spaces, infusing the surroundings with a soft and inviting glow. Scents like lavender, eucalyptus, or sandalwood offer a comforting and calming atmosphere, making guests feel more at ease and enhancing their overall well-being.

When hosting guests, offering scented towels infused with essential oils is a luxurious touch that immediately conveys a sense of hospitality and care. Warm or cool towels infused with refreshing scents like peppermint or citrus oils provide a stimulating and invigorating welcome. This simple yet impactful gesture engages the senses, awakening and energizing guests upon arrival. The aromatic towels serve a practical purpose and set the stage for a positive and memorable experience, signaling to guests that their comfort and enjoyment are a top priority.

Furthermore, incorporating essential oils into the linens and bedding enhances the restful quality of guest accommodations. A light misting of a linen spray infused with oils like lavender or chamomile adds a touch of luxury to the sleeping environment. These calming scents contribute to a more restful night's sleep, promoting relaxation and helping guests unwind after a day of activities or travel. This approach is especially beneficial in hospitality settings, such as hotels or bed and breakfasts, where the quality of the sleeping environment plays a crucial role in guest satisfaction.

In spa or wellness settings, where relaxation is the primary focus, essential oils create an immersive and soothing experience for guests. Aromatherapy massage, for instance, combines the therapeutic benefits of touch with the calming effects of essential oils. Blends tailored to individual preferences or wellness goals, such as stress relief or muscle relaxation, enhance the overall massage experience. The carefully chosen scents contribute to the sensory enjoyment of the treatment and complement the therapeutic effects, creating a holistic and rejuvenating experience for guests.

Beyond individual treatments, spa environments can benefit from the diffusion of essential oils throughout the facility. A consistent and harmonious aromatic theme, such as a lavender, geranium, and cedarwood blend, can be diffused in common areas, treatment rooms, and relaxation spaces. This cohesive approach ensures guests are enveloped in a continuous and immersive aromatic journey from entering the spa. Essential oils in spa settings extend to steam rooms, saunas, and relaxation lounges, where carefully selected scents contribute to the overall sense of tranquility and rejuvenation.

For those hosting gatherings at home, creating a welcoming and relaxing environment for guests involves a combination of thoughtful touches and strategic use of essential oils. A bowl of potpourri infused with aromatic oils placed in the entryway or living room provides a delightful and lasting impression. Potpourri allows for a customizable and decorative display of dried flowers, herbs, and botanicals infused with essential oils, emitting a subtle and continuous fragrance throughout the space. The visual appeal of potpourri, coupled with the pleasing scents, enhances the overall ambiance and sets the stage for a warm and inviting atmosphere.

In addition to diffusers, candles, and scented towels, incorporating essential oils into culinary and beverage offerings further enriches the guest experience. Aromatic herbs and citrus oils can be incorporated into dishes and drinks, tantalizing the taste buds while complementing the sensory experience. For example, a refreshing glass of infused water with slices of citrus fruits and a hint of mint can be a delightful and hydrating welcome for guests. Similarly, incorporating essential oils into recipes for appetizers or desserts adds a unique and flavorful element to the dining experience, aligning the aromatic journey with culinary enjoyment.

When crafting a relaxing environment for guests, it is essential to consider individual preferences and sensitivities. Opting for universally appealing scents, such as lavender or citrus, ensures that the aromatic experience is enjoyable for diverse individuals. Providing options for personalization, such as offering a selection of diffuser blends or scented towels with different oils, adds a thoughtful and inclusive element to the experience. The goal is to create a space that invites guests to unwind, connect, and fully engage in the celebratory or hospitable atmosphere.

In conclusion, the strategic use of essential oils in creating a relaxing environment for guests elevates the overall experience, making it memorable, enjoyable, and rejuvenating. Whether diffused in communal areas, incorporated into spa treatments, or infused into culinary offerings, essential oils create a multisensory experience that engages and delights guests. The artful combination of visual, tactile, and aromatic elements sets the stage for an environment where guests feel welcomed, cared for, and able to immerse themselves fully in the celebratory or hospitable atmosphere.

Using Essential Oils in Meditation and Reflection

Incorporating essential oils into meditation and reflection practices has gained widespread popularity, offering individuals a powerful and aromatic tool to deepen their spiritual experiences. The synergy between essential oils and mindfulness practices, such as meditation and reflection, creates a unique sensory experience that enhances the journey inward, fostering a sense of tranquility, focus, and connection. Whether used in diffusers, applied topically, or inhaled directly, essential oils can elevate these practices' spiritual and contemplative aspects, guiding individuals on a transformative and aromatic journey.

Diffusing essential oils during meditation serves as an effective means to create an ambient and supportive atmosphere. The gentle dispersion of aromatic molecules into the air engages the olfactory senses, instantly transforming the meditation space into a sanctuary of scents. A carefully chosen blend of essential oils, such as frankincense, lavender, and sandalwood, can induce a state of calmness and relaxation, easing the transition into a meditative state. The aromatic backdrop is a subtle anchor, helping practitioners center their thoughts and emotions and facilitating a more profound and focused meditation experience.

Selecting essential oils with grounding and centering properties aligns with the objectives of meditation and reflection. Earthy scents like patchouli and vetiver or woody aromas like cedarwood and pine evoke a sense of rootedness and stability. These oils provide a supportive foundation for meditation, helping individuals feel more connected to the present moment and grounded in their contemplative practice. The grounding qualities of these oils assist in quieting the mind, reducing distractions, and fostering a more profound sense of inner peace.

In addition to diffusion, the direct inhalation of essential oils can be a potent method for enhancing meditation and reflection. A drop or two of a chosen oil applied to the palms gently rubbed together, and cupped over the nose allows for intentional and controlled inhalation. This direct connection with the essence of the oil intensifies the sensory experience, creating a more immediate and personal connection with the chosen aroma. Whether focusing on a single oil or creating a synergistic blend, inhaling essential oils becomes integral to the breathwork and mindfulness exercises associated with meditation.

Applying essential oils topically during meditation involves diluting them with a carrier oil and gently massaging the blend onto specific pulse points or body areas. This method allows for a more intimate and tactile experience with the oils, encouraging a deeper integration of their aromatic properties. Oils such as lavender or chamomile, known for their calming and soothing effects, can be applied to the wrists, temples, or neck to promote relaxation and create a sensory connection to the meditation practice. Self-massage with essential oils becomes a ritualistic and self-nurturing aspect of the meditative journey.

Essential oils can also be incorporated into meditation by creating personalized blends tailored to specific intentions or themes. For example, if the goal is to enhance spiritual connection, a blend of oils with sacred and uplifting properties, such as frankincense, myrrh, and sandalwood, can be crafted. Similarly, for those seeking clarity and focus during meditation, invigorating oils like peppermint, eucalyptus, or rosemary may be included in the blend. The intentional selection and blending of oils align with the reflective aspects of meditation, allowing individuals to infuse their practice with a personalized aromatic signature.

The transformative potential of essential oils in meditation extends to supporting individuals in navigating emotional landscapes and promoting emotional well-being. Essential oils with calming and emotionally balancing properties, such as bergamot, clary sage, or ylang-ylang, can be particularly beneficial for those using meditation for introspection and self-awareness. The gentle aroma of these oils helps create a space where emotions can be explored with a sense of calmness and acceptance, fostering a more compassionate and open-hearted meditative experience.

Beyond their impact on the sensory aspects of meditation, essential oils hold significance in various spiritual and cultural traditions. Many ancient practices, such as Ayurveda and traditional Chinese medicine, incorporate aromatic substances for spiritual and healing purposes. Oils like frankincense and myrrh, revered for their sacred qualities, have been used for centuries in rituals and ceremonies to evoke a sense of reverence and connection to the divine. Incorporating these oils into meditation can resonate with these historical and spiritual traditions, deepening the sense of sacredness within the contemplative practice.

Moreover, using essential oils in meditation aligns with the principles of holistic well-being, acknowledging the interconnectedness of the mind, body, and spirit. As individuals engage in meditation to cultivate inner peace, clarity, and spiritual connection, the aromatic support of essential oils becomes a natural extension of this holistic approach. The oils contribute to a harmonious and integrated experience, bridging the realms of the physical and the metaphysical and fostering a sense of unity within the self.

Practitioners of meditation and reflection often find that creating a dedicated and intentional space for their practice enhances its effectiveness. This includes considerations for lighting, comfort, and, notably, aromatics. The careful selection of essential oils allows individuals to curate an environment that resonates with their intentions and facilitates a seamless transition into a meditative state. Whether through the ceremonial application of oils, the aromatic ambiance of diffusion, or the symbolic use of sacred scents, essential oils become an integral part of the holy space, elevating the meditative experience.

In conclusion, using essential oils in meditation and reflection represents a harmonious union of aromatic alchemy and spiritual practice. Whether diffused, inhaled, applied topically, or integrated into personalized blends, essential oils contribute to an inward multi-sensory journey, enhancing meditation's transformative and contemplative aspects. The intentional selection and use of oils align with the goals of mindfulness, creating an environment that fosters tranquility, presence, and connection to the self. As individuals embark on their aromatic meditative journeys, essential oils' subtle yet profound influence becomes a guiding force, supporting them in exploring the depths of their inner landscapes and spiritual consciousness.

CHAPTER X
Beyond the Basics: Deepening Your Understanding

Resources for Further Learning

Embarking on a journey into the world of essential oils invites individuals to explore aromatic wonders and holistic well-being. As enthusiasts delve into the vast and intricate landscape of essential oils, it becomes crucial to have access to reliable resources that provide comprehensive information, guidance, and ongoing education. Fortunately, a wealth of resources is available, catering to beginners and seasoned practitioners. These resources encompass books, online courses, reputable websites, and expert-led workshops, collectively offering a rich tapestry of knowledge that empowers individuals to deepen their understanding of essential oils and their diverse applications.

Books are foundational resources for those seeking a comprehensive understanding of essential oils. Renowned authors in the field, such as Robert Tisserand, Valerie Ann Worwood, and Kurt Schnaubelt, have penned authoritative works that cover necessary oil basics, therapeutic applications, and safety guidelines. Tisserand's "Essential Oil Safety" is considered a definitive guide on the safe use of essential oils, offering insights into potential contraindications and proper dilution practices. Worwood's "The Complete Book of Essential Oils and Aromatherapy" is a comprehensive guide for beginners and advanced practitioners, delving into the therapeutic properties of various oils and providing practical applications. Schnaubelt's "The Healing Intelligence of Essential Oils" explores the profound healing potential of essential oils, merging scientific understanding with holistic approaches.

Online courses have become invaluable for individuals seeking a structured and interactive learning experience. Platforms like Aromahead Institute, The School for Aromatic Studies, and NAHA (National Association for Holistic Aromatherapy) offer courses catering to various expertise levels. Aromahead Institute, founded by Andrea Butje, provides a range of courses, from foundational aromatherapy to advanced blending techniques. The School for Aromatic Studies, led by Jade Shutes, offers in-depth courses on topics like aromatherapy for the immune system and clinical aromatherapy. NAHA provides many resources, including webinars and educational events, fostering a sense of community among aromatherapy enthusiasts. These online courses impart knowledge and facilitate a dynamic and interactive learning environment, allowing participants to engage with experts and fellow learners.

Reputable websites and online platforms dedicated to aromatherapy serve as valuable hubs for ongoing learning and exploration. The National Association for Holistic Aromatherapy (NAHA) website and its educational offerings provide a wealth of articles, research papers, and safety guidelines, making it a go-to resource for aromatherapy enthusiasts. AromaWeb, curated by aromatherapist Wendy Robbins, offers an extensive array of articles, recipes, and essential oil profiles, catering to beginners and advanced practitioners. Important Oil University, founded by Dr. Robert Pappas, is a reputable source for in-depth scientific information about essential oils, including detailed chemical profiles and analytical reports. These online platforms serve as virtual libraries, offering a plethora of information that spans the spectrum of necessary oil knowledge.

Expert-led workshops and seminars provide an immersive and hands-on learning experience, allowing participants to deepen their understanding under the guidance of experienced practitioners. Aromatherapy conferences, such as the International Federation of Professional Aromatherapists (IFPA) and the Alliance of International Aromatherapists (AIA), bring together experts worldwide, offering workshops, lectures, and networking opportunities. Local aromatherapy associations and schools often host workshops featuring renowned educators, allowing participants to engage directly with experts and enhance their practical skills. These workshops offer valuable insights and foster a sense of community among enthusiasts, creating spaces for shared experiences and knowledge exchange.

Podcasts have emerged as a convenient and accessible medium for learning about essential oils, featuring expert interviews, discussions on specific topics, and practical tips for enthusiasts. Podcasts like "The Essential Oil Revolution," hosted by Samantha Lee Wright, and "Aromatic Wisdom" by Liz Fulcher, delve into various aspects of aromatherapy, providing a blend of practical advice and expert insights. These podcasts offer a convenient way for individuals to stay informed, especially for those with busy schedules or those who prefer audio-based learning. Listening to discussions and interviews with experts adds a dynamic and engaging dimension to the learning experience, making complex concepts more accessible.

Journals and research publications are indispensable resources for those interested in the scientific aspects of essential oils. The Journal of Essential Oil Research, published by Taylor & Francis, features peer-reviewed articles on essential oils' chemistry, pharmacology, and therapeutic applications. PubMed, a biomedical literature database, is a valuable resource for accessing scientific studies related to essential oils. Exploring these scholarly sources provides a more in-depth understanding of various essential oils' biochemical composition and potential therapeutic effects, bridging the gap between traditional knowledge and contemporary scientific research.

Social media platforms offer vibrant communities where individuals can connect with fellow enthusiasts, share experiences, and learn from one another. Facebook groups, Instagram accounts, and forums dedicated to aromatherapy provide spaces for discussions, recipe sharing, and troubleshooting common challenges. Engaging with these online communities allows individuals to tap into the collective wisdom of a diverse group of aromatherapy practitioners. It also provides an avenue for seeking advice, sharing success stories, and staying updated on the latest trends and developments in the field.

In conclusion, learning about essential oils is enriched by a diverse array of resources catering to different learning preferences and levels of expertise. Books, online courses, reputable websites, expert-led workshops, podcasts, research publications, and social media communities collectively form a robust ecosystem that empowers individuals to explore, understand, and integrate the art and science of aromatherapy into their lives. As the field continues to evolve, these resources serve as beacons of knowledge, guiding enthusiasts on a perpetual journey of discovery and holistic well-being through the captivating world of essential oils.

Advanced Applications of Essential Oils

The world of essential oils, with its rich tapestry of aromas and therapeutic properties, extends beyond basic applications, inviting enthusiasts to explore advanced and nuanced approaches. As practitioners delve deeper into the intricacies of essential oils, they uncover a myriad of advanced applications that go beyond conventional uses. From specialized therapeutic blends to synergistic formulations for emotional well-being, the advanced realm of essential oil applications unveils a holistic and sophisticated approach to harnessing the full potential of these aromatic essences.

One advanced application of essential oils lies in therapeutic blending, where practitioners skillfully combine multiple oils to create synergistic effects tailored to specific health concerns. Blending essential oils is an art that involves a deep understanding of the therapeutic properties, chemical constituents, and energetics of each oil. For example, creating a blend for respiratory support might apply combining oils with expectorant properties, such as eucalyptus and tea tree, with anti-inflammatory oils like frankincense. The precise combination of oils in therapeutic blends amplifies their benefits, creating a powerful and targeted remedy for various health conditions.

In emotional well-being, advanced applications of essential oils extend to creating intricate blends designed to address specific emotional states and promote psychological balance. Practitioners leverage the profound impact of aromas on the limbic system, which is intricately linked to emotions and memory. Blends crafted for emotional support often include oils known for calming, uplifting, or grounding properties. For instance, a blend for stress relief might incorporate lavender, bergamot, and chamomile to soothe the nervous system and induce a sense of tranquility. The artful formulation of these blends allows individuals to navigate the complexities of emotions and promote a harmonious balance between the mind and spirit.

Advanced applications also encompass essential oils in energetic and spiritual practices. Many ancient traditions recognize the spiritual significance of aromatic substances, using them to enhance meditation, rituals, and energetic healing. Oils like frankincense, myrrh, and sandalwood hold historical and symbolic importance and are often associated with sacred ceremonies and spiritual awakening. Practitioners may incorporate these oils into meditation practices, energy-clearing rituals, or ceremonies, tapping into the subtle energies of the oils to deepen their spiritual connection and foster a sense of transcendence.

Aromatherapy massage, an advanced application of essential oils, involves the skillful integration of oils into therapeutic massage sessions. Beyond the necessary dilution for skin safety, practitioners consider the specific therapeutic objectives of the massage and tailor their oil selection accordingly. For example, a massage to alleviate muscle tension may involve using oils with analgesic and anti-inflammatory properties, such as peppermint and lavender. Combining skilled massage techniques and the targeted application of essential oils enhances the overall therapeutic experience, promoting relaxation, pain relief, and emotional well-being.

Essential oils find advanced applications in skincare formulations designed for specific skin concerns and conditions. Practitioners and skincare experts craft blends that address acne, aging, and inflammation. Oils like tea tree, rosehip, and helichrysum may be combined to create potent blends with antimicrobial, regenerative, and anti-inflammatory properties. The advanced use of essential oils in skincare involves a nuanced understanding of skin types, sensitivities, and the compatibility of various oils with different cosmetic bases. These carefully formulated blends offer a natural and holistic approach to promoting skin health and radiance.

Furthermore, the advanced applications of essential oils extend to pain management. Practitioners may develop specialized blends for targeted relief from various types of pain, including headaches, muscle aches, and joint discomfort. Oils such as peppermint, eucalyptus, and ginger are known for their analgesic and anti-inflammatory properties, making them valuable components of pain-relieving formulations. The synergy created by combining these oils allows for a more comprehensive and practical approach to managing pain, offering individuals natural alternatives to conventional remedies.

In advanced aromatherapy practices, essential oils are harnessed for their psychotherapeutic effects, playing a role in addressing emotional and psychological challenges. Aromatherapists may work with clients to create personalized blends that support mental health, addressing issues like anxiety, depression, or insomnia. Oils with adaptogenic properties, like lavender and bergamot, are often incorporated to help individuals adapt to stressors and find emotional balance. The therapeutic relationship between aromatherapist and client becomes a collaborative journey, utilizing the nuanced effects of essential oils to promote mental well-being.

Neuroaromatherapy is an advanced application exploring the direct impact of essential oils on the brain and nervous system. This field delves into the intricate relationship between aromatic compounds and neurotransmitters, examining how specific oils influence mood, cognition, and overall brain function. For instance, inhaling citrus oils like lemon or orange has been associated with increased alertness and improved mood, making them valuable tools in promoting cognitive function. Neuroaromatherapy explores the potential of essential oils as natural interventions for mental clarity, focus, and emotional resilience.

Advanced applications of essential oils also extend to the creation of natural perfumery, where skilled artisans blend oils to craft personalized and complex fragrances. Unlike commercial perfumes that often contain synthetic chemicals, natural perfumery relies on the intricate aromas of essential oils to create unique and captivating scents. Perfumers consider the top, middle, and base notes of oils and their olfactory profiles and synergies. This artful blending allows individuals to wear fragrances that appeal to their sense of smell and offer therapeutic benefits, contributing to a sensory experience that aligns with their personal well-being.

The realm of advanced applications in essential oils includes the exploration of their antiviral, antibacterial, and antifungal properties. Practitioners may develop potent formulations for immune support, environmental cleansing, or personal hygiene. Oils like tea tree, thyme, and oregano are known for their antimicrobial effects, making them valuable additions to formulations designed to combat pathogens. Advanced aromatherapists consider the scientific research behind the antimicrobial properties of essential oils and apply this knowledge to create effective and natural alternatives for maintaining a healthy and clean environment.

In conclusion, the advanced applications of essential oils represent a sophisticated and multifaceted exploration of their therapeutic potential. From therapeutic blending and emotional well-being to energetic practices and skincare formulations, practitioners delve into essential oils' nuanced art and science. The versatility of these aromatic essences allows for a holistic approach to well-being, addressing physical, emotional, and spiritual aspects. As individuals and practitioners continue to deepen their understanding and refine their skills, the advanced applications of essential oils unveil a vast and captivating terrain, inviting exploration, creativity, and a profound connection with the transformative power of aromatherapy.

Becoming an Informed Consumer

Becoming an informed consumer of essential oils is an empowering journey that involves acquiring knowledge, discernment, and a critical understanding of the market. Essential oils derived from plant sources have gained immense popularity for their therapeutic and aromatic properties. Still, the vast and diverse market offers a range of products that vary in quality, purity, and ethical considerations. To navigate this landscape effectively, consumers must equip themselves with the tools to make informed choices, ensuring they receive the benefits of authentic and high-quality essential oils while avoiding potential pitfalls.

One fundamental aspect of being an informed consumer is understanding the concept of purity in essential oils. Pure essential oils are extracted solely from the botanical source, free from synthetic additives, diluents, or contaminants. However, the market is rife with products labeled as "essential oils" that may be diluted with carrier oils or synthetic substances. Reading product labels is crucial in discerning an essential oil's purity. Genuine essential oils typically list the botanical name, indicating the specific plant from which the oil is derived. Furthermore, reputable manufacturers provide information about the extraction method, ensuring transparency about the oil's production process.

The sourcing and cultivation of plants for essential oil production play a pivotal role in determining the quality of the final product. Informed consumers prioritize oils sourced from reputable and ethical producers who adhere to sustainable and environmentally friendly practices. Ethical considerations extend to factors such as fair trade practices, ensuring that local communities involved in the cultivation and harvesting of plants receive fair compensation for their labor. Consumers contribute to a more sustainable and socially responsible essential oil industry by choosing oils from conscientious producers.

Understanding the concept of therapeutic grade, a term often used in the essential oil market, is another aspect of informed consumption. It is important to note that there is no universally accepted standard for a therapeutic grade, and the term is frequently used as a marketing tool. Reputable essential oil companies, however, adhere to high-quality standards and provide information about their testing processes. Informed consumers seek oils that undergo rigorous testing for purity, potency, and authenticity. Third-party testing by independent laboratories adds a layer of credibility, ensuring that the essential oil meets the specified quality standards.

One of the primary factors influencing the quality of essential oils is the extraction method employed during production. Informed consumers familiarize themselves with various extraction methods, such as steam distillation, cold pressing, and CO_2 extraction, each with nuances and impact on the final product. Steam distillation, for instance, is a standard method that preserves the delicate aromatic compounds of the plant. Cold pressing is suitable for citrus oils, while CO_2 extraction is known for producing oils with a broader spectrum of aromatic components. Awareness of extraction methods empowers consumers to choose oils that align with their preferences and therapeutic needs.

A critical aspect of becoming an informed consumer is recognizing red flags and avoiding common pitfalls in the essential oil market. For instance, claims that an essential oil can cure specific diseases or ailments should be met with skepticism. While essential oils have therapeutic properties, they should not be considered a substitute for professional medical advice or treatment. Informed consumers prioritize safety and consult healthcare professionals when needed, especially if they have pre-existing health conditions or are considering essential oils for specific therapeutic purposes.

Additionally, price can indicate quality in the essential oil market. While high-quality oils may come with a higher price tag due to factors such as plant scarcity, responsible sourcing, and meticulous production processes, consumers should be cautious of meager prices. Meager prices may signal poor quality, adulteration, or unethical sourcing practices. Informed consumers recognize the value of investing in high-quality essential oils for a more authentic and practical aromatic experience.

Researching and staying informed about reputable essential oil brands is critical to responsible consumption. Informed consumers seek brands that prioritize transparency, providing detailed information about their sourcing, testing, and production practices. Trustworthy brands readily share information about the origins of their oils, cultivation methods, and ethical considerations. Engaging with customer reviews, testimonials, and expert recommendations can also guide consumers toward reputable brands with a track record of delivering high-quality essential oils.

The concept of impurity is a significant concern in the essential oil market, highlighting the importance of being an informed consumer. Adulteration involves diluting or altering crucial oils with synthetic additives, compromising their purity and therapeutic properties. Informed consumers educate themselves about common adulterants and employ methods to detect potential signs of impurity. For example, gas chromatography-mass spectrometry (GC-MS) testing is a reliable technique used by reputable manufacturers to analyze the chemical composition of essential oils, ensuring their authenticity.

Engaging with educational resources is a proactive step for consumers seeking to deepen their understanding of essential oils. Reputable books, online courses, and workshops led by experienced aromatherapists provide valuable insights into the world of essential oils. Learning about the botanical profiles, therapeutic properties, and safe usage guidelines enhances consumers' decision-making. Educational resources also empower consumers to explore the diverse applications of essential oils, from aromatherapy and massage to skin care and emotional well-being.

Informed consumers recognize the importance of proper storage and handling to preserve the integrity of essential oils. Heat, light, and air exposure can degrade the quality of oils over time. Dark glass bottles, preferably amber or cobalt blue, protect oils from light exposure, while airtight seals prevent oxidation. Proper storage in a cool, dark place helps maintain the stability and longevity of essential oils, ensuring that consumers receive the full spectrum of aromatic and therapeutic benefits.

Ultimately, becoming an informed consumer of essential oils is a dynamic and ongoing process involving curiosity, education, and discernment. As consumers equip themselves with knowledge about purity, sourcing, extraction methods, and potential pitfalls, they navigate the market with confidence. Informed consumers prioritize authenticity, quality, and ethical considerations, contributing to a sustainable and conscientious essential oil industry. This journey of informed consumption not only enhances the aromatic experiences of individuals but also supports a responsible and transparent marketplace for crucial oils.

CONCLUSION

In conclusion, "Oil of Life: A Comprehensive Beginner's Guide to Essential Oils - Harnessing the Power of Nature for Everyday Well-Being" stands as a beacon of enlightenment for those venturing into the world of essential oils. This e-book expertly navigates the intricate realm of aromatherapy, distilling complex information into an accessible and comprehensive guide for beginners. From the origins and extraction processes of essential oils to their diverse therapeutic applications, the e-book weaves together a tapestry of knowledge that empowers readers to harness the transformative power of nature for their everyday well-being.

The e-book's chapter-based format systematically explores essential oils, covering their types, extraction methods, and various applications. "Oil of Life" strikes a perfect balance by offering in-depth information without overwhelming the reader, making it an invaluable resource for those stepping into aromatherapy for the first time. The emphasis on safety measures, including proper dilution and usage guidelines, ensures that readers can fully enjoy the benefits of essential oils while respecting their potency.

Throughout its pages, the e-book imparts practical knowledge and cultivates an appreciation for the holistic benefits of essential oils. From their potential in skincare routines to their role in creating relaxing atmospheres, the guide encourages readers to integrate these natural wonders seamlessly into their daily lives.

"Oil of Life" does more than educate; it inspires a newfound appreciation for the gifts of nature and encourages a shift towards holistic well-being. By demystifying essential oils and offering practical insights, the e-book provides a solid foundation for individuals embarking on their journey with these aromatic wonders. Whether readers seek stress relief, enhanced mood, or natural remedies for various ailments, this guide equips them with the tools to harness the therapeutic potential of essential oils.

In essence, "Oil of Life" is not just a guide but a

companion on the path to well-being. As readers delve into the world of essential oils through the pages of this e-book, they find themselves on a transformative journey, discovering the art and science of aromatherapy and unlocking the power of nature to enhance their everyday lives.

Thank you for buying and reading/listening to our book. If you found this book useful/helpful please take a few minutes and leave a review on the platform where you purchased our book. Your feedback matters greatly to us.

www.ingramcontent.com/pod-product-compliance
Lightning Source LLC
LaVergne TN
LVHW012024060526
838201LV00061B/4450